Cambridge Elements ≡

Elements in High-Risk Pregnancy: Management Options
edited by
David James
University of Nottingham
Philip Steer
Imperial College London
Carl Weiner
Creighton University School of Medicine
Stephen Robson
Newcastle University

DIABETES IN PREGNANCY

Lee Wai Kheong Ryan
KK Women's and Children's Hospital, Singapore

Lim Weiying
Singapore General Hospital, Singapore

Ann Margaret Wright
KK Women's and Children's Hospital, Singapore

Lay-Kok Tan
KK Women's and Children's Hospital, Singapore

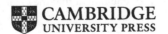

CAMBRIDGE
UNIVERSITY PRESS

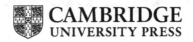

CAMBRIDGE
UNIVERSITY PRESS

Shaftesbury Road, Cambridge CB2 8EA, United Kingdom

One Liberty Plaza, 20th Floor, New York, NY 10006, USA

477 Williamstown Road, Port Melbourne, VIC 3207, Australia

314–321, 3rd Floor, Plot 3, Splendor Forum, Jasola District Centre,
New Delhi – 110025, India

103 Penang Road, #05–06/07, Visioncrest Commercial, Singapore 238467

Cambridge University Press is part of Cambridge University Press & Assessment,
a department of the University of Cambridge.

We share the University's mission to contribute to society through the pursuit of
education, learning and research at the highest international levels of excellence.

www.cambridge.org
Information on this title: www.cambridge.org/9781009507158

DOI: 10.1017/9781009507189

When citing this work, please include a reference to the DOI 10.1017/9781009507189

First published 2025

A catalogue record for this publication is available from the British Library

ISBN 978-1-009-50715-8 Paperback
ISSN 2976-8330 (online)
ISSN 2976-8322 (print)

Diabetes in Pregnancy

Elements in High-Risk Pregnancy: Management Options

DOI: 10.1017/9781009507189
First published online: January 2025

Lee Wai Kheong Ryan
KK Women's and Children's Hospital, Singapore

Lim Weiying
Singapore General Hospital, Singapore

Ann Margaret Wright
KK Women's and Children's Hospital, Singapore

Lay-Kok Tan
KK Women's and Children's Hospital, Singapore

Author for correspondence: Lee Wai Kheong Ryan, rylee82@yahoo.com

Abstract: Diabetes mellitus is one of the most common and important medical complications affecting pregnancy. It can predate the pregnancy ('pre-existing diabetes') or arise during pregnancy ('gestational diabetes', GDM). Typically, GDM resolves once the pregnancy has ended. However, about 3% of women with a diagnosis of GDM have type 2 diabetes diagnosed for the first time in pregnancy, which persists beyond pregnancy. The co-existence of diabetes of any type and pregnancy is associated with an increased risk of adverse outcomes for both the woman and baby. However, with appropriate management by a multidisciplinary team before, during and after delivery these risks can be minimised. Optimising blood glucose control, screening for maternal and fetal complications and a discussion about delivery are key strategies. During pregnancy, all women should be offered screening for GDM. After pregnancy, all women with GDM should be offered annual screening to identify the development of type 2 diabetes.

Keywords: pregnancy, diabetes, high risk, management, multidisciplinary

ISBNs: 9781009507158 (PB), 9781009507189 (OC)
ISSNs: 2976-8330 (online), 2976-8322 (print)

Contents

Commentary

Diabetes mellitus is one of the most common and important medical complications affecting pregnancy. The number of pregnant women with diabetes is rising worldwide.

Diabetes can pre-date the pregnancy ('pre-existing diabetes') or arise during pregnancy ('gestational diabetes', GDM). Typically, GDM resolves once the pregnancy has ended. However, about 3% of women with a diagnosis of GDM actually have type 2 diabetes diagnosed for the first time in pregnancy and therefore it persists after the pregnancy is over. About 30% of women with GDM will develop type 2 diabetes within 10 years, and up to 50% over a longer period.

The coexistence of diabetes of any type and pregnancy is associated with an increased risk of adverse outcomes for both the woman and the baby, in particular macrosomia and resulting difficulties at delivery (such as shoulder dystocia). However, with appropriate management by a multidisciplinary team before, during and after delivery these risks can be minimised. Women with pre-existing diabetes should be counselled before pregnancy about the implications of pregnancy, and given particular support to optimise blood glucose control and the management of related medical complications when trying to conceive.

During pregnancy, women should be offered screening for GDM. This can be either 'universal' in which all pregnant women are screened, or only those with 'risk factors', such as a body mass index (BMI) >30, previous gestational diabetes or macrosomia, or a first-degree relative with diabetes. Screening for GDM is only for women not known to have a diagnosis of diabetes.

Women with either pre-existing diabetes or GDM require multidisciplinary care during the pregnancy. Assiduous blood glucose monitoring is essential to allow adjustment of medication with the aim of achieving blood glucose values within the normal range. Pregnancy is a diabetogenic state and in known pre-existing diabetes more insulin or oral hypoglycaemic medication will be needed. The closer maternal blood glucose values are to normal, the lower the likelihood of adverse outcomes in the woman and the baby. In addition, women are offered medications to lessen the likelihood of complications; for example, low-dose aspirin to reduce the risk of pre-eclampsia in the woman, and folic acid to reduce the risk of neural tube defects in the fetus. Apart from aiming for optimal blood glucose control, women should be monitored for the complications of the diabetes. Fetal assessment in the pregnancy includes accurate ultrasound measurements, especially in the first trimester to optimise dating of the pregnancy and throughout pregnancy, screening for fetal abnormality and ongoing surveillance of fetal growth, placenta function and amniotic fluid volume.

Every woman with diabetes in pregnancy should be offered a delivery plan discussion. This covers the timing and method of delivery, which are influenced by factors including the quality of blood glucose control and the presence of maternal and/or fetal complications. Irrespective of the method of delivery, caregivers should aim to maintain normal glucose values. In labour, a continuous glucose and insulin infusion will best maintain glucose homeostasis, and the fetal heart rate should be continuously monitored.

After delivery, blood glucose levels in women with pre-existing diabetes usually return to pre-pregnancy values, and most women with GDM will have normal blood glucose values with treatment. However, about 3% will need ongoing care of their diabetes, usually in the form of oral hypoglycaemic agents. All women with GDM should be offered annual screening for diabetes to identify the development of type 2 diabetes.

For at least the first 72 hours after the delivery, the baby should receive close surveillance for and treatment of possible complications, hypoglycaemia in particular.

Despite the progress made in the understanding, screening and management of gestational diabetes and pre-existing diabetes in pregnancy, controversies remain, which is evident in differing professional society guidelines. For example, although there is agreement that treatment of GDM has benefits, there is a still a lack of a clear threshold for increased risk of adverse pregnancy outcomes, which was made very clear by the Hyperglycaemia and Adverse Pregnancy Outcomes (HAPO) study, which demonstrated that the association between maternal plasma glucose concentrations (for both fasting and post-glucose challenge values) and adverse pregnancy outcomes is linear and continuous, with no inflection point.

Furthermore, there is no good evidence to support treatment of GDM at International Association of Diabetes and Pregnancy Study Group (IADPSG) thresholds. The inevitable additional diagnoses of GDM based on IADPSG thresholds increases the burden of diagnosis to both patients and the healthcare system. Finally, although it is recommended that women with GDM get tested for type 2 diabetes six weeks postnatally, the reality is that many women do not attend this testing and alternative approaches are needed. Not surprisingly, this current situation has left healthcare providers without consensus guidelines, resulting in the variability in care for GDM.

Another inherent problem is the definition of GDM, " ... any degree of glucose intolerance of onset or first detected in pregnancy irrespective of whether the condition persists after pregnancy (and) does not exclude the possibility that (it) antedated pregnancy". This definition conflates trivial increases in maternal glucose with overt but previously unrecognised diabetes (usually type 2) and wrongly implies that the risks are the same across this spectrum. The woman with unrecognised diabetes has significant adverse outcomes (congenital anomalies and stillbirth) compared to the true GDM patient. In communities with a high local prevalence of type 2 diabetes and obesity having the condition being detected first during pregnancy is not uncommon, and screening strategies for early pregnancy detection are needed.

More research is therefore needed to progress from the current broad agreement that pregnant women should be screened for GDM towards reaching consensus on optimal screening, diagnostic criteria, treatment, or post-delivery screening.

1 Introduction

Diabetes mellitus is one of the most common and important medical complications affecting pregnancy [1,2]. The rising prevalence and burden of diabetes worldwide has led to an increasing number of women being affected by pre-existing diabetes mellitus in pregnancy and gestational diabetes mellitus (GDM) [3,4].

2 Epidemiology

The prevalence of diabetes mellitus worldwide has been steadily increasing in recent years, in part due to the rising average body mass index (BMI) [5,6]. In addition, women have also been deferring childbirth till later in life, which has led to an increased incidence of cases of both pre-existing diabetes in pregnancy and GDM. There are also changing thresholds to defining GDM and differing screening practices exist. It is estimated that diabetes mellitus affects about 1 in 6 (17%) pregnancies. Of these, about 14% had pre-gestational diabetes and 86.4% have GDM [7].

3 Pathophysiology

The fetoplacental unit requires glucose as the main energy substrate. As fetal gluconeogenesis is minimal, the fetus is dependent on placental glucose transfer via glucose transporter proteins (GLUTs). Maternal insulin sensitivity varies over the course of the pregnancy (see Figure 1) [8]. Peak insulin sensitivity occurs between 9 and 16 weeks' gestation, which predisposes insulin-treated women to hypoglycaemia. Thereafter, insulin resistance and insulin requirements continue to rise, with a peak and then plateau at around 36 weeks' gestation. Insulin resistance increases in pregnancy due to placental hormones, including human placental lactogen, progesterone, prolactin, placental growth hormone and cortisol. Increasing insulin resistance is associated with compensatory hyperinsulinaemia in non-diabetic pregnancy. In women with pre-existing diabetes mellitus, the compensatory rise in endogenous

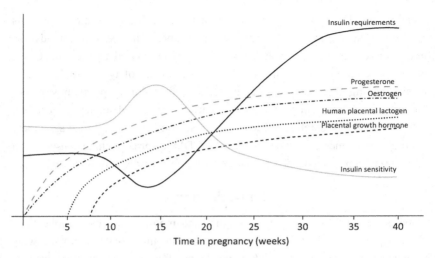

Figure 1 Insulin requirements and sensitivity throughout pregnancy [8].

insulin production does not occur, with resultant greater maternal hypergly-caemia, especially postprandial.

In addition, pregnancy is a state of 'accelerated starvation', where there is an exaggerated response to overnight fasting compared to the non-pregnant state. This means there is a greater fall in plasma glucose and amino acids, and a more pronounced rise in free fatty acids with enhanced ketogenesis during periods of fasting during pregnancy [9].

4 Classification of Diabetes in Pregnancy

Pregnancy can be affected by either pre-existing diabetes (DM) or gestational diabetes mellitus (GDM), which is diagnosed in pregnancy.

Pre-existing Diabetes Mellitus

Pre-existing diabetes mellitus is defined as women who have either type 1 or type 2 diabetes and less commonly maturity-onset diabetes of the young (MODY) before pregnancy. Glucokinase (GCK) MODY (MODY 2) or hepatocyte nuclear factor 1a (HNF1a) MODY (MODY 3) are the two most common types of MODY. Glucokinase MODY is an interesting condition, as the pregnancy outcome is dependent on the fetal carrier status for GCK mutation (50%), where fetuses without the GCK mutation are at higher risk of macrosomia. As such, regular fetal growth assessment can help establish appropriate glucose targets for women with known or suspected GCK mutations. Other less-common causes of DM include pancreatitis and iatrogenic diabetes secondary to medications such as glucocorticoids and antiretroviral therapy.

Gestational Diabetes Mellitus

Gestational diabetes mellitus has been defined as any degree of glucose intolerance with onset or first recognition during pregnancy. It may reflect previously undiagnosed pre-existing diabetes. Women with GDM have at least a sevenfold increased risk of developing DM in the future [10]. Because of the increasing worldwide prevalence of undiagnosed type 2 diabetes mellitus in non-pregnant women of childbearing age, several screening algorithms, based on expert consensus, have been advocated to identify women with pre-existing diabetes which is first detected during pregnancy to differentiate them from true gestational diabetics [11,12,13]. This has clinical implications, because the risk profiles for the two groups are different. Women with pre-existing diabetes are more likely to develop microvascular complications such as retinopathy and nephropathy [14,15,16] and are at increased risk of congenital malformations associated with pre- compared with gestational diabetes [17,18].

5 Maternal, Fetal and Neonatal Risks of Diabetes in Pregnancy

Diabetes in pregnancy is associated with increased risks of adverse maternal, fetal and neonatal outcomes during pregnancy (Table 1) [8]. These correlate largely with maternal glycaemic control [19,20]. Whereas many of the risks of diabetes in pregnancy are common across all types of diabetes, women with type 1 and type 2 diabetes mellitus face additional risks, such as increased risk of congenital malformations, stillbirth, severe hypoglycaemia, diabetic ketoacidosis and worsening of existing microvascular disease [21,22]. Screening for GDM in pregnancy is important because of the higher risk of complications in pregnancy as well as long-term cardiometabolic complications [2,22].

The rates of pregnancy loss from miscarriage for both type 1 and type 2 DM are similar, but the risk factors differ, with losses in type 1 DM most commonly being attributable to major congenital anomaly and prematurity, whereas for type 2 it is stillbirth and chorioamnionitis [23,24]. Pregnant women with pre-existing diabetes are more likely to develop microvascular complications such as nephropathy and retinopathy, which can worsen during pregnancy [15]. The incidences of diabetic nephropathy in women with type 1 and type 2 diabetes are reported as 5–10% and 2–3%, respectively [15,16]. Diabetic retinopathy affects almost 50% of women with type 1 and 14% with 2 diabetes [25].

Table 1 Adverse pregnancy outcomes associated with diabetes in pregnancy [8]

Maternal	Fetal	Neonatal
• Hypoglycaemia • Diabetic ketoacidosis • Pregnancy-induced hypertension and pre-eclampsia • Diabetes-related complications (retinopathy, nephropathy)[#] • Perineal lacerations • Operative vaginal delivery • Caesarean section • Postpartum haemorrhage • Infection • Risk of DM with history of GDM[*]	• Miscarriage • Intrauterine death • Stillbirth • Congenital malformations[#] • Intrauterine growth restriction • Fetal macrosomia	• Preterm delivery • Shoulder dystocia • Birth injuries • Hypoglycaemia • Polycythaemia • Hyperbilirubinaemia • Hypocalcaemia • Respiratory distress syndrome • Obesity and metabolic syndrome in the future

*Risks unique to GDM; [#]risks unique to pre-existing DM.

6 Management Options for Diabetes in Pregnancy

Pre-pregnancy (Women with Pre-existing Diabetes)

General

Preconception care should be part of the routine care for all women of reproductive age with pre-existing diabetes. It should be provided by a multidisciplinary team comprising an obstetrician, endocrinologist, specialised diabetes nurse and dietician who should provide women with knowledge and advice to optimise their health for the best outcomes when they become pregnant.

A recent UK National pregnancy in Diabetes Audit report 2020 [26] recommends:

• Having dedicated pre-pregnancy coordinators focusing on pre-conception preparations, such as enhancing provision of contraception and folic acid administration, and the improvement of glycaemic control, especially in women with pre-existing diabetes living in deprived regions. Pregnancy preparation rates are lowest in women from the most deprived communities – only

6% of women with type 2 diabetes and 21% with type 1 diabetes living in areas with the lowest quintiles of deprivation were prepared for pregnancy as per NICE (National Institute for Health and Care excellence) guidelines.

- Enhancing access to structured education, weight management and diabetes prevention programmes for women with previous gestational and early-onset type 2 diabetes should be prioritised.

Various pre-pregnancy programmes, such as the community pre-pregnancy care (PPC) programme advocated by Murphy et al., have been shown to improve pregnancy outcomes and reduce adverse outcomes in women with pre-existing diabetes [27,28] with consequential healthcare cost savings [21,29]. The above-mentioned pre-pregnancy care programme encompassed the use of patient information leaflets for all eligible women with pre-existing diabetes mellitus, provision of preconception care templates for use during primary care consults and provision of online PPC education modules.

Pre-pregnancy Counselling

The American Diabetes Association recommends that prenatal counselling should be part of routine diabetes care for all women of reproductive age [30]. Critical aspects of this counselling include:

- Highlighting the importance of planning pregnancy to optimise diabetes control, detect and treat diabetes-related complications.
- Advising of the increased risks associated with unplanned pregnancy including the risk of congenital malformations.
- Offering contraceptive advice and family planning during diabetic stabilisation.
- Reviewing the patient's medication to ensure drug safety for pregnancy.
- Stressing the importance of preconceptual high-dose folic acid (5 mg) daily to reduce the risk of neural tube defects ideally at least three months before conception and continued until the end of first trimester.

Apart from counselling, pre-pregnancy care of women actively planning pregnancy should include:

- Monitoring glycaemic control
- Review and optimisation of medication
  - o Optimisation of glucose-lowering medications
  - o Cessation/substitution of potentially teratogenic medications
  - o Folic acid supplementation
- Screening for and management of diabetes-related complications

o Diabetic retinopathy
o Diabetic nephropathy
o Cardiovascular disease
• Assessment and management of coexisting medical conditions
o Hypertension
o Hyperlipidaemia
o Thyroid disorders
• Nutrition and weight management

Glycaemic Control

Strict glycaemic control is crucial for planned pregnancy as periconception maternal hyperglycaemia is associated with a higher risk of miscarriage [1,19] congenital malformation, stillbirth and neonatal death [31,32].

The aim is to minimise fetal exposure to maternal hyperglycaemia during the period of fetal organogenesis, which occurs prior to seven weeks' gestation, which is often before a woman finds out she is pregnant [33]. Periconception glycaemic control has been reported as an independent predictor of congenital malformation with a 1% (11 mmol/mol) linear increase in glycated haemoglobin (HbA1c) above 6.3% (45 mmol/mol) [31]. Most international bodies (Table 2) recommend a preconception HbA1c target of <48 mmol/mol or <6.5%, as this is associated with risk of congenital anomalies equivalent to the non-diabetic population [31,34].

Evidence is scarce regarding target capillary glucose or interstitial glucose levels for women planning pregnancy. The 2015 NICE guidelines recommend that women with pre-existing DM who are planning pregnancy should aim for the same capillary blood glucose (CBG) targets as those for all patients with type 1 DM [36]. These are a fasting level of 5–7 mmmol/l and levels of 4–7 mmol/l pre-meal and 5–9 mmol/l at least 90 min post-meal [36].

Optimising Medication for Pre-pregnancy

Oral Glucose-lowering Medications

The two main oral glucose-lowering medications used for pre-pregnancy and during pregnancy are metformin and glibenclamide (glyburide). The recommendations by various international groups for the use of oral glucose lowering agents in pregnancy vary considerably [41]. The American Diabetes Association (ADA) recommends converting oral agents to insulin therapy as a preferred management strategy [30]. The National Institute for Health and Care Excellence recommends that metformin may continue to be used as an adjunct or alternative to insulin, when the potential benefits of improved glycaemia outweigh the risk of harm, and also

Table 2 Preconception glycaemic targets for pregnancy
from international guidelines

Guideline	HbA1c (mmol/mol, %)	Fasting/ pre-meal glucose (mmol/l)	Postprandial glucose (mmol/l)
American Diabetes Association (2020) [30]	<48, 6.5	Nil	Nil
Diabetes Canada Clinical Practice Guidelines Expert Committee (2018) [35]	≤48, 6.5	Nil	Nil
The National Institute for Health and Care Excellence (NICE) (2015) [36]	<48, 6.5	5–7 mmol/l on waking 4–7 mmol/l before meals at other times of the day	5–9 mmol/l at least 90 min postprandially
The Endocrine Society (2013) [37]	Aim for HbA1c levels as close to normal as possible when they can be safely achieved without undue hypoglycaemia	≤5.3 mmol/l	1 h after the start of a meal: ≤7.8 mmol/l 2 h after the start of a meal: ≤6.7 mmol/l

recommends ceasing all other blood glucose-lowering agents [42]. Diabetes Canada recommends continuing metformin and/or glibenclamide if glycaemic control is optimal until conception, whereas women on other agents should be switched to insulin therapy [35]. There are insufficient data on other oral glucose-lowering drugs (α-glucosidase inhibitors, thiazolidinediones, dipeptidyl peptidase-4 (DPP-4) inhibitors, and sodium-glucose cotransporter-2 (SGLT-2) inhibitors) to justify their use in human pregnancy.

Metformin is a biguanide that decreases blood glucose levels by reducing hepatic glucose output and increasing insulin sensitivity. Its use is associated with a lower risk of hypoglycaemia or weight gain, as there is no stimulation of insulin secretion from the pancreas. Metformin crosses the placenta readily and metformin levels in the fetal circulation have been reported to be between half and the same as the maternal metformin levels [41,43]. The data regarding the short-term safety of metformin use in both early and late pregnancy are reassuring. Several meta-analyses have shown no evidence for an increased risk of major malformations and adverse neonatal outcomes with first-trimester metformin use [44,45,46]. However, there is limited long-term follow-up information, especially concerning metformin use in pregnancies complicated by pre-existing diabetes. The MiG-TOFU study, conducted in Australia and New Zealand, evaluated metabolic outcomes for children born to 751 women with GDM randomly allocated at 20–33 weeks to receive either open treatment with either metformin (with added insulin if needed to control blood glucose values) or insulin [47]. At age seven, 290 children from the Australian cohort were assessed and there were no differences in offspring measures of body composition among the insulin and metformin subgroups. At age nine, 99 children from the New Zealand cohort were reviewed. Although the children in the metformin subgroup were larger than the insulin subgroup by measures of weight, arm and waist circumferences, waist: height ($p < 0.05$), BMI, triceps skin fold (p: 0.05), DEXA fat mass and lean mass (p: 0.07), their body fat percentage was similar by DEXA and bioimpedance [48]. Their visceral adipose tissue and liver fat were similar by magnetic resonance imaging (MRI). Metabolic markers including HbA1c, fasting glucose, fasting lipids, adiponectin and leptin were all similar.

Glibenclamide (glyburide) is a second-generation sulfonylurea that lowers blood glucose levels by enhancing the release of insulin from β cells in the pancreatic islets in response to stimulation by glucose. Glibenclamide can be added if a woman does not attain optimal glucose targets on metformin and declines insulin treatment, or if she is intolerant of metformin. In the MiG-TOFU trial, up to 50% of women on metformin therapy required supplementary insulin later in pregnancy [47]. Similarly, glibenclamide appeared to have a therapy failure rate of 20%, with these women requiring insulin therapy [49].

Insulin

Insulin formulations that are approved for use in pregnancy include human insulin [neutral protamine Hagedorn (NPH) insulin and regular insulin], insulin aspart and lispro (both rapid-acting insulin analogues), and insulin detemir (long-acting insulin analogue).

Insulin-treated women with diabetes planning to get pregnant should be treated with multiple daily insulin injections (MDIIs) or a continuous subcutaneous insulin infusion (CSII), as these regimens are more likely than premixed insulin therapy to achieve target blood glucose levels during the preconception period and during pregnancy. Multiple daily insulin injection therapy involves the use of intermediate- or long-acting basal insulin to inhibit hepatic glucose production and lipolysis throughout the day and mealtime short- or rapid-acting insulin to cover dietary carbohydrate intake. Continuous subcutaneous insulin infusion therapy involves the continuous infusion of rapid-acting insulin by an insulin pump.

Until the 1980s, animal insulin (derived from cows and pigs) was the only treatment for insulin-dependent diabetes. Their use has now been almost entirely replaced by synthetic human insulin and human analogue insulin (analogue insulins are very similar to human insulin, but they have one or two amino acids changed. Analogue insulin preparations have been modified to change how fast and how slow they act after injection). Soluble (regular) insulin is a quick-acting human insulin formulation, which has a slower onset and a longer duration of action than endogenous insulin. This confers an increased risk of undesirable postprandial hypoglycaemia [50]. (Rapid-acting insulin analogues include lispro, aspart, and glulisine). These can be used as mealtime insulin in MDII therapy or in an insulin pump. Rapid-acting insulin analogues have faster onset of action, earlier time to peak, and shorter duration of action than regular insulin, mimicking endogenous insulin physiology more closely. This allows rapid-acting insulin analogues to provide superior control of postprandial hyperglycaemia and reduce risks of hypoglycaemia.

Long-acting insulin analogues include detemir and glargine. Detemir has been approved for use by the European Medicines Agency and the U.S. Food and Drug Administration (FDA) for use in pregnancy. Some women may require twice-daily dosing of detemir due to interindividual variability in the duration of action. Limited data on the glargine use in women with pre-existing DM suggest comparable maternal, fetal and neonatal outcomes compared with other basal insulins [51–53]. Insulin glargine does not carry an FDA classification consistent with current labelling. However, the Endocrine Society in the USA and NICE in the UK have suggested that women whose diabetes is well controlled with insulin glargine prior to pregnancy may continue to use this insulin analogue before and during gestation [37,54].

Lee et al. showed that hybrid closed-loop insulin therapy significantly improved maternal glycaemic control during pregnancy complicated by type 1 diabetes mellitus. Compared to standard care using multidose insulin therapy, the closed-loop group had lower HbA1c levels, reduced time spent in hyperglycaemia, and higher overnight time in target range. Hybrid closed-loop insulin pump use may be the way forward for type 1 diabetes mellitus in pregnancy [55].

Cessation/Substitution of Potentially Teratogenic Medications

Women should stop any potentially teratogenic medications before conception, and they should be replaced by safer alternative medications at, or as soon as possible after, confirmation of pregnancy. Drugs that should be avoided include angiotensin-converting enzyme (ACE) inhibitors (ACE-I), angiotensin receptor blockers (ARB), and statins.

Folic Acid Supplementation

Women with pre-existing diabetes should receive folic acid supplementation at least 1–3 months prior to conception to reduce the risk of neural tube defects [56]. Although not evidence-based, a higher dose (5 mg/day) is sometimes recommended for women with diabetes and should be given until week 12 of gestation (36).

Screening and Management of Diabetes-related Complications

a. Diabetic Retinopathy

Women should undergo retinal examination prior to conception to determine the presence and severity of diabetic retinopathy (DR) [30]. Ophthalmologist referral should be made if severe non-proliferative diabetic retinopathy (NPDR), proliferative diabetic retinopathy (PDR), or diabetic macular oedema are detected. Women should be advised about the risks of worsening retinopathy during and up to 1 year after pregnancy, especially if severe [57,58]. Overall, 10–26% of women without retinopathy will develop background retinopathy changes during pregnancy. However, these are generally mild, do not require intervention and usually regress postpartum [59,60]. However, if surgery is required, the Endocrine Society recommends deferring conception until the retinopathy has been treated and stabilised [37].

b. Diabetic Nephropathy

Women embarking on a pregnancy should be screened for diabetic nephropathy (DN) with measurement of serum creatinine and evaluation of albuminuria with a spot urine albumin-to-creatinine ratio (ACR) or a 24-hour urinary protein measurement. Women with a serum creatinine ≥120 μmol/l, urine ACR >30 mg/mmol or estimated glomerular filtration rate (eGFR) <45 ml/min should see a nephrologist before discontinuation of contraception. In women with more advanced renal dysfunction, pregnancy may lead to permanent worsening of renal function and accelerate progression to end stage renal failure. These women need to be extensively and sensitively counselled regarding the possibility of renal dialysis or future transplant prior to, or even during, pregnancy.

Evidence of ACE-I and ARB teratogenicity for first-trimester exposures is conflicting and usage during pregnancy is not recommended as fetal renin angiotensin aldosterone blockade may result in renal failure, oligohydramnios, fetal growth restriction (FGR), and fetal death [61,62]. Enalapril and captopril are considered compatible with breastfeeding by the American Academy of Pediatrics and may be restarted after delivery [63].

c. Cardiovascular Disease

Women who have symptoms or history of ischaemic heart disease should be referred to a cardiologist prior to withdrawal of contraception. Pregnancy is contraindicated with severe cardiac disease such as Marfan's syndrome with aortic root diameter >4.5 cm, severe symptomatic aortic stenosis, severe mitral stenosis and coarctation of aorta with aneurysm [64].

Assessment and Management of Coexisting Medical Conditions

a. Hypertension

Most guidelines recommend a blood pressure target of <135/85 mmHg for women with pre-existing diabetes [42,65,66]. Blood pressures lower than 120/80 mmHg should be avoided because they can result in reduced fetal growth.

b. Hyperlipidaemia

Women with pre-existing diabetes may have metabolic syndrome–related hyperlipidaemia. Statins are not recommended for use during pregnancy. It is unlikely that withdrawing statins for the limited duration of conception, pregnancy and breastfeeding will have significant long-term adverse health outcomes for the mother [30,37]. Women who have significant hypertriglyceridaemia [raised triglyceride (TG) levels] should receive dietary counselling encouraging them to have a low-fat diet with less than 20% of calories from fat. Omega-3 fatty acids (3–4 g per day) lower TG levels and prevent essential fatty acid deficiency, which may arise from a fat-restricted diet [67]. Routine use of fibrates and niacin during pregnancy is not recommended [37].

c. Thyroid Disorders

Autoimmune thyroid disease such as Hashimoto thyroiditis and Graves' disease occur more frequently in women with type 1 DM (T1DM). Women with T1DM wanting to conceive should have their serum thyroid stimulating hormone (TSH) measured before planning for pregnancy. Thyroid peroxidase antibodies (TPOAb) should be measured if not done previously. Women with T1DM are also more prone to postpartum thyroid dysfunction, with an incidence of 25% [68]. They should be screened for postpartum thyroiditis with serum TSH measurements at 3 and 6 months postpartum [37].

Nutrition and Weight Management

Obesity is common in patients with type 2 DM (T2DM+), and increasingly prevalent in patients with T1DM [69]. Dietary therapy should be individualised based on the woman's BMI and degree of physical activity [70]. Caloric restriction may be necessary to prevent excessive weight gain and aid glycaemic control in women with GDM. In addition, a targeted calorie-controlled low-glycaemic index (GI) diet is recommended as it results in less-frequent use of insulin and lower birth weights when compared with control diets [71]. Physical activity improves insulin sensitivity [72] and women with no contraindications should aim to accumulate at least 150 min of moderate-intensity physical activity each week to reduce the risk of pregnancy complications [73].

Prenatal (Women with Pre-existing Diabetes and Gestational Diabetes)

Women with diabetes in pregnancy should be encouraged to be involved in their pregnancy care under the management of the multidisciplinary team of health-care professionals.

Screening for Gestational Diabetes and Blood Glucose Control

Screening For and Diagnosis of Diabetes in Pregnancy

Published guidelines differ in their recommendations for both screening and diagnosis (see Table 3).

Screening can be either of the whole population ('universal') or only those women 'at risk'. For universal screening, either sequential or one-step testing may be used. The most common investigation for sequential testing is the non-fasting 50-g, 1-hour glucose challenge test (GCT) at 24–28 weeks' gestation [77]. A woman who is screened positive using the 50-g GCT will then be subject to confirmation testing via a full oral glucose tolerance test (OGTT), either the 100-g 3-h OGTT or, in some units, the 75-g 2-h OGTT. In the one-step approach, a fasting 75-g OGTT is performed at 24–28 weeks' gestation [77]. Risk-based screening can unfortunately miss cases of GDM in women with no

Table 3 Summary of different diagnostic criteria for GDM diagnosis

Organisation	WHO 2013 [74]	IADPSG 2010 [75]	ACOG 2018 [63]	Canadian Diabetes Association 2018 [76]	ADA 2020 [30]	NICE 2015 [36]
Screening	Women with risk factors	All	Women with risk factors	All	All	Women with risk factors
Screen method	1 step 75 g	1 step 75 g	50 g glucose challenge test (GCT)	50 g GCT	1 step 75 g	1 step 75 g
Screen +ve	N/A	N/A	≥7.8	≥7.8	N/A	N/A
Oral glucose tolerance test	75 g	75 g	100 g	75 g	75 g	75 g
Fasting (mmol/L)	≥5.1	≥5.1	≥5.3	≥5.1	≥5.1	≥5.6
1 h (mmol/L)	≥10.0	≥10.0	≥10.0	≥10.6	≥10.0	–
2 h (mmol/L)	≥8.6	≥8.5	≥8.6	≥9.0	≥8.5	≥7.8
3 h (mmol/L)	–	–	≥7.8	–	–	–

risk factors [78] when compared to universal screening, which will identify nearly all women with GDM. Published series suggest that, depending on the risk factors used, their definition (for example, BMI weight threshold or previous baby weight threshold) and the population being studied, risk factor screening could result in sensitivities of 93–100% and specificities of 4–32%. Opting for risk-factor screening rather than universal screening is usually decided on the basis of cost and available resources.

As an example of risk-based screening, the 2015 NICE guidelines recommend selective screening for GDM using the following risk factors at the booking appointment [36]:

- BMI > 30 kg/m^2
- having a previous baby weighing ≥ 4,500 g
- history of previous GDM
- family history of diabetes (first-degree relative)
- minority ethnic family origin with a high prevalence of diabetes

The NICE guideline recommends that women with one or more of these risk factors should be offered a formal 75-g 2-h OGTT. If the results of the OGTT are normal, the woman should be offered a repeat 75-g 2-h OGTT at 24–28 weeks.

In 2010, the IADPSG proposed new diagnostic criteria for GDM based on a graded dose–response, associating maternal glycaemia with the pregnancy outcomes reported in the HAPO study [79]. The HAPO study showed that glucose intolerance in pregnancy is a continuum, so the higher the glucose level, the higher the risk of adverse outcomes [73]. The HAPO study showed a continuous positive linear relationship between maternal fasting and 1- and 2-h plasma glucose levels on the OGTT, and failed to identify a diagnostic glucose threshold. The IADPSG diagnostic thresholds were the glucose values at which the odds for adverse outcomes (birth weight, C-peptide concentration and percentage of newborns with neonatal body fat greater than the 90th centile) reached 1.75 times the odds of these outcomes at the mean glucose values of the entire study cohort deemed not to have pre-existing diabetes mellitus [79]. The IADPSG recommended that GDM be diagnosed if one or more of the following criteria are met:

- fasting plasma glucose ≥ 5.1 mmol/l
- 1-h plasma glucose ≥ 10.0 mmol/l following a 75-g oral glucose load
- 2-h plasma glucose ≥ 8.5 mmol/l following a 75-g oral glucose load

In 2013, the World Health Organisation (WHO) endorsed and adopted the IADPSG diagnostic criteria for GDM in an attempt to achieve universal diagnostic criteria for GDM. Similarly, the IAPDSG criteria have since been adopted by several organisations such as the American Diabetes Association [30], the Australasian Diabetes in Pregnancy Society (ADIPS) [80], the International Federation of Gynecology and Obstetrics (FIGO) [81] and Sweden [82].

Glycaemic Targets and Monitoring

Women are more insulin-sensitive in the first trimester, but become increasingly insulin-resistant in the second and third trimesters [83]. Summarised data from 11 studies evaluating third-trimester glucose levels of non-diabetic pregnant women suggests that the fasting glucose is 3.1–4.9 mmol/l (95% CI), 1 h postprandial is 5.3–6.8 mmol/l (95% CI) and 2 h postprandial glucose is 4.9–6.1 mmol/l (95% CI) [84]. Currently, there are no adequately powered randomised controlled trials (RCTs) evaluating the impact of different glycaemic targets for diabetes in pregnancy. Targets recommended by various guidelines are summarised in Table 4. Most of these targets are extrapolated from studies evaluating normoglycaemia in pregnancy, and pregestational and gestational DM [85,86,87].

Capillary Blood Glucose Monitoring

Regular self-monitoring of blood glucose (SMBG) is essential for titration of DM treatment in pregnancy. SMBG should be performed preprandial, postprandial (1 or 2 h after the start of a meal) and at bedtime. Postprandial glucose is superior to preprandial glucose as a predictor of fetal macrosomia [94,95,96].

The timing of postprandial glucose checks should ideally capture peak postprandial glucose levels. A study utilising continuous glucose monitoring demonstrated that the average peak postprandial glucose level occurs 90 min after a meal, with significant variation between individuals [97]. Multiple factors contribute to this, such as variable gastric emptying, meal timings, glycaemic index or macronutrient content of meals [98,99,100].

The need for frequent finger pricks for capillary blood glucose (CBG) monitoring is cumbersome and painful. Newer methods of glucose monitoring involve measurement of the interstitial fluid glucose via continuous glucose monitoring (CGM) and flash glucose monitoring systems [101]. However, these technologies are more costly and not all have been validated for use in pregnancy. Continuous glucose monitoring devices measure interstitial glucose at 5–10-s intervals, providing about 288 values per day [101]. There are two types of CGM, real-time and retrospective CGM. Glucose sensors for CGM devices typically last for a week, and generally at least two CBG readings per day are required for sensor calibration. CGM may identify glucose excursions that go undetected by CBG testing [97,98,102].

Table 4 Summary of target glucose and HbA1c levels for pre-existing diabetes
in pregnancy from international guidelines

Guideline	Fasting/ preprandial (mmol/l)	1-h postprandial (mmol/l)	2-h postprandial (mmol/l)	HbA1c (mmol/mol, %)
The American College of Obstetricians and Gynaecologists (ACOG) 2018 [65]	<5.3	<7.8	<6.7	<42, 6.0
American Diabetes Association (ADA) 2020 [30]	<5.3	<7.8	<6.7	<42, 6.0
The National Institute for Health and Care Excellence (NICE) 2015 [36]	<5.3	<7.8	<6.4	<48, 6.5
Australasian Diabetes in Pregnancy Society (ADIPS) (2005) [80]	≤5.5	≤8.0	≤7.0	<42, 6.0
Diabetes Canada Clinical Practice Guidelines Expert Committee (2018) [76]	<5.3	<7.8	<6.7	<48, 6.5 (first and second trimester) <43, 6.1 (third trimester)

In the planning pregnancy arm of the landmark Continuous Glucose
Monitoring in Pregnant Women with Type 1 Diabetes Trial (CONCEPTT)
[38], it was found that there were no significant benefits for CGM for women
with T1DM. This contrasts with the pregnant arm, where CGM use resulted in
small improvements in HbA1c, greater time-in-target, fewer hypoglycaemic

episodes and better neonatal outcomes [38]. At present, CGM has been recommended for pregnant women with type 1 diabetes [39]. Evidence of clinical effectiveness and cost-effectiveness for women with type 2 diabetes mellitus or GDM has not yet been established.

More data are needed to evaluate whether widening access to technologies such as Libre [40] (a flash glucose monitor, which uses a sensor that is placed on the back of the upper arm and worn externally by the user, allowing glucose information to be monitored using a mobile app when it is passed over the sensor) or a CGM (which can be connected to an insulin infusion pump as part of a closed-loop feedback control system) will result in improved control of glucose levels during the second and third trimesters, especially among pregnant women with type 2 diabetes [39].

The Abbott Freestyle Libre flash glucose monitoring system (flash-GMS) similarly measures interstitial fluid glucose. A reader or smartphone is used to scan a glucose sensor worn on the back of the arm. There is no need for calibration with CBG readings, and the sensor lasts for up to 14 days [103,104]. Flash-GMS is not approved for use in pregnancy in most countries [105,106]. The accuracy of flash-GMS compared to CBG is acceptable with the mean absolute difference at 11.8% [92,107]. However, there are concerns regarding accuracy of flash-GMS in pregnancy, with readings having a tendency to be lower than CBG readings, which may result in divergent treatment decisions [92]. There are no available RCTs to validate the use of flash-GMS in pregnancy.

The ADA recommended that CGM should not be used as a replacement for CBG monitoring but rather as a supplementary modality of glycaemic monitoring [30]. The use of flash-GMS in pregnancy is not currently advocated by any guideline.

Glycated Haemoglobin

In the non-pregnant state, HbA1c reflects average blood glucose concentrations during the preceding 12 weeks [108]. In pregnancy, there is increased red cell turnover, which lowers HbA1c [109]. HbA1c may therefore be monitored more frequently during pregnancy due to increased red cell turnover, for example once every 4 weeks to access glycaemic control [110]. The limitation of HbA1c monitoring is that it cannot reveal the degree of glycaemic variability, or postprandial hyperglycaemia, which drives macrosomia [111]. Therefore, self-monitoring of blood glucose is the primary method of glucose monitoring in pregnancy [30].

- Elevated first-trimester HbA1c is associated with poor outcomes such as stillbirth, spontaneous abortion and congenital abnormalities (see Figure 2)

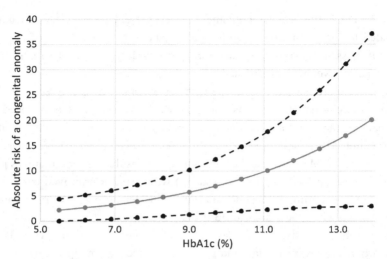

Figure 2 Absolute risk of a major or minor congenital anomaly according to
periconceptional HbA1c. Data presented as absolute risk
(solid line) and ±95% CIs (dashed lines).

Adapted from Guerin A, Nisenbaum R, Ray JG. Use of maternal GHb concentration to estimate the risk of congenital anomalies in the offspring of women with
pre-existing diabetes in pregnancy. *Diabetes Care.* 2007;30:1920–25. (113)

[34,112,113]. Elevated third-trimester HbA1c at or above 48 mmol/mol or
6.5% is associated with macrosomia, preterm delivery and pre-eclampsia
[112,114]. Most guidelines suggest an HbA1c target of <6.0–6.5%
[76,80,115]. While striving for these tight targets, avoidance of hypoglycaemia remains important due to associated risks of low birth weight, in
addition to the usual risks of hypoglycaemia [116].

Pharmacotherapy

Women with pre-existing diabetes should receive treatment with oral glucose-
lowering agents and/or insulin. Women with type 1 diabetes mellitus are
dependent on exogenous insulin therapy whereas women with type 2 diabetes
mellitus or GDM may be offered oral agents or insulin. As discussed above in
the pre-pregnancy section, the two main oral glucose-lowering agents used in
pregnancy are metformin and glibenclamide (glyburide). The ADA [30] recommends converting oral agents to insulin therapy as a preferred management
strategy. NICE [42] recommends that metformin may continue to be used as an
adjunct or alternative to insulin when the potential benefits of improved glycaemia outweigh the risk of harm.

Adjuvant Therapies for Women with Diabetes in Pregnancy

Aspirin for Pre-eclampsia Prevention

Pre-eclampsia is a multisystem disorder of pregnancy, usually defined as hypertension and proteinuria diagnosed after 20 weeks' gestation. Women with pre-existing DM have an increased risk of pre-eclampsia. Women with longer histories of DM and vascular complications have a further increased risk [117,118]. Low-dose aspirin (80–150 mg) reduces the risk of pre-eclampsia when initiated before 16 weeks gestation and taken throughout pregnancy [119].

Folic acid

As discussed above, women with pre-existing diabetes should receive folic acid supplementation to reduce the risk of neural tube defects [55,56]. Although not evidence-based, a higher dose (5 mg/day) is sometimes recommended for women with diabetes and should be given until week 12 of gestation [36].

Lifestyle Management and Medical Nutrition Therapy

Medical Nutrition Therapy

Nutrition therapy is the cornerstone of DM management and all individuals with DM in pregnancy should be referred to a registered dietitian for individualised medical nutritional therapy. The goals are to provide enough nutrients for mother and fetus, achieve optimal weight gain and maintain ideal glycaemic control.

There is no optimal diet for diabetes in pregnancy. The Institute of Medicine (IOM) has suggested an approximate macronutrient distribution for all populations comprising 40–60% carbohydrates, 30% protein and 10% fats. The minimum carbohydrate requirements increase in pregnancy from 130 g/day to 175 g/day [120]. Carbohydrate requirements should be individualized based on weight gain targets, insulin doses, glucose readings and patient preference. Carbohydrates that have low GI are preferred to improve postprandial glycaemic control [121].

Weight Management

Overweight or obese women who experience pregnancy weight gain greater than IOM recommendations have more adverse outcomes, including increased macrosomia and higher rates of Caesarean deliveries [122,123]. Although not specific to women with pre-existing diabetes, IOM guidelines recommend

Table 5 2009 Institute of Medicine Recommendations
for Weight Gain During Pregnancy [124]

Pre-pregnancy BMI	Total weight gain		Rates of weight gain in second and third trimesters	
	Range (kg)	Range (lb)	Mean weight gain (range), kg/week	Mean weight gain (range), lb/week
Underweight (<18.5 kg/m^2)	12.5–18	28–40	0.51 (0.44–0.58)	1 (1–1.3)
Normal weight (18.5–24.9 kg/m^2)	11.5–16	25–35	0.42 (0.35–0.50)	1 (0.8–1)
Overweight (25.0–29.9 kg/m^2)	7–11.5	15–25	0.28 (0.23–0.33)	0.6 (0.5–0.7)
Obese (≥30.0 kg/m^2)	5–9	11–20	0.22 (0.17–0.27)	0.5 (0.4–0.6)

weight gain in pregnancy based on a woman's pre-pregnancy weight or BMI (Table 5).

Weight loss is not recommended during pregnancy because of potential adverse fetal outcomes. All weight loss efforts in women who are overweight with BMI ≥27 kg/m^2 [36] should take place prior to conception and reasonable realistic targets set to reduce adverse outcomes. Weight loss in pregnancy is not recommended as it is associated with fetal growth restriction.

Exercise

Low to moderate exercise during pregnancy has been found to improve glycaemic control among women with gestational diabetes and appears safe with no reports of maternal or neonatal complications (125) Pregnant women with no contraindications should aim to accumulate at least 150 min of moderate-intensity physical activity each week to reduce the risk of pregnancy complications (73).

Organisation of Prenatal Care

Women should ideally have received pre-pregnancy counselling and women with pre-existing diabetes should be seen by a joint diabetes and obstetric team as soon as possible when they become pregnant [39]. Table 6 shows a suggested antenatal care schedule for women with diabetes.

Table 6 Suggested schedule of prenatal care for women with diabetes

Gestational age	Pre-existing diabetes	Gestational diabetes
Booking appointment (joint diabetes and antenatal care) as soon as possible after informing professionals they are pregnant	Emphasise importance of optimal blood glucose control and dietary advice Establish extent and severity of diabetes-related complications Review medications Retinal and renal assessment if these have not been done in the previous year Measure HbA1c levels to ascertain level of risk for the pregnancy Confirm viability of pregnancy and gestation age	Offer self-monitoring of blood glucose or a 75-g OGTT for women with a history of GDM if booked in the first trimester If GDM is diagnosed in the first trimester, follow advice given under pre-existing diabetes
16 weeks	Offer retinal assessment if retinopathy was present at the first visit	Offer self-monitoring of blood glucose or a 75-g OGTT for women with a history of GDM if booked in the second trimester
20 weeks	Ultrasound scan to screen for structural anomalies and examination of the four-chamber view of the fetal heart and outflow tracts	If GDM is diagnosed in the first or second trimester, ultrasound scan to screen for structural anomalies and examination of the four-chamber view of the fetal heart and outflow tracts
28 weeks	Ultrasound monitoring of fetal growth and amniotic fluid volume Retinal assessment if not previously done	Those diagnosed at 24–28 weeks should be referred to the National Diabetes Prevention Programme if eligible Ultrasound monitoring of fetal growth and amniotic fluid volume

Table 6 (cont.)

Gestational age	Pre-existing diabetes	Gestational diabetes
32 weeks	Ultrasound monitoring of fetal growth and amniotic fluid volume	
34 weeks	No additional or different care from non-diabetic pregnancies	
36 weeks	Ultrasound monitoring of fetal growth and amniotic fluid volume Discuss timing, mode, and management of birth Discuss analgesia and anaesthesia, and changes to blood glucose therapy during and after birth, care of the neonate, breastfeeding, contraception, and follow-up	Ultrasound monitoring of fetal growth and amniotic fluid volume
37 weeks	Offer induction of labour for poorly controlled diabetes or if fetal complications occur, or Caesarean section for obstetric indications	Offer induction of labour for poorly controlled GDM, or Caesarean section for obstetric indications; otherwise await spontaneous onset of labour, if well controlled on dietary therapy
38 weeks	Offer induction of labour or Caesarean section for obstetric indications	Offer tests of fetal well-being
39 weeks		Advise women with uncomplicated GDM to deliver no later than 40^{+6} weeks

(Adapted from NICE, Diabetes in Pregnancy QS 109 [39])

Maternal Surveillance and Management

Maternal Complications

Diabetic Retinopathy

As indicated above all women should have pre-pregnancy retinal evaluation performed. Ideally patients should be monitored every trimester and for one year postpartum as indicated by the degree of retinopathy [30]. Pan-retinal laser photocoagulation may be used safely and effectively for treatment of PDR during pregnancy [126]. Anti-VEGF medications (Ranibizumab, Aflibercept and Bevacizumab) are used for treatment of diabetic macular oedema (DME) in non-pregnant patients. However, these agents have been assigned FDA pregnancy category C and there are no controlled data in human pregnancy, so a risk–benefit approach needs to be taken regarding their use [127]. Background retinopathy changes may occur during pregnancy, but these are usually mild.

Diabetic Nephropathy

Baseline renal function including creatinine and albumin creatinine ration should have been established pre-pregnancy as mentioned above. Blood pressure control using agents which are safe in pregnancy is important for the management of DN during pregnancy. Blood pressure-lowering therapy should be started if the blood pressure consistently exceeds 135/85 mmHg. Blood pressure targets should not be lower than 120/80 mmHg, as this may impair fetal growth [30]. Safe and effective antihypertensive agents, which can be substituted for ACE inhibitors and angiotensin receptor blockers while actively planning or during pregnancy, include methyldopa, nifedipine, labetalol, hydralazine, diltiazem, prazosin, and clonidine [30,37].

There is no guidance on the schedule of care for women with chronic kidney disease, but renal function should be monitored regularly antenatally and in the postpartum period. One suggested approach is to monitor serum creatinine and urine albumin/creatinine ratio at least 4 weekly, and at least fortnightly from 32 weeks' gestation [128].

Hypertension

Hypertensive disorders in pregnancy are common in women with diabetes. Type 1 diabetes is more often associated with pre-eclampsia, whereas T2DM is more often associated with chronic hypertension [129]. Most guidelines recommend a blood pressure target of <135/85 mmHg for women with pre-existing diabetes [65,66,76]. Pressures lower than 120/80 mmHg should be avoided as they are associated with fetal growth restriction.

Pre-eclampsia

In a retrospective study of 1,813 women with GDM, the incidence of pre-eclampsia was higher in women with fasting plasma glucose ≥5.8 mmol/l (13.8%) than in those with fasting plasma glucose <5.8 mmol/l (7.8%) [130]. The rate of pre-eclampsia in GDM women has been found to be more than double the rate in non-diabetic women (6.1% vs. 2.8%) and has been found to be influenced by the severity of GDM [131]. Symptoms and signs of pre-eclampsia should be sought at every visit after 20 weeks given the higher risk of those with both GDM and pre-existing DM [132,133,134]. Those with pre-existing hypertension, nephropathy, and/or a previous history of pre-eclampsia are at particular risk.

Diabetic Ketoacidosis in Pregnancy

Diabetic ketoacidosis (DKA) in pregnancy is associated with 4–15% maternal and 10–35% neonatal mortality [135,136]. Due to constant transplacental transfer of glucose and nutrients, DKA in pregnancy may present atypically with euglycaemic DKA [137].

Physiological changes in pregnancy increase susceptibility to DKA. First, in pregnancy, fat breakdown, ketosis and protein catabolism occur more quickly. Second, there is a reduced buffering capacity in view of increased alveolar minute ventilation, with resultant compensatory increase in renal excretion of bicarbonate. Lastly, the presence of diabetogenic hormones such as human placental lactogen, free cortisol, prolactin and progesterone results in increased insulin resistance [138]. The usual precipitants for DKA are sepsis, intercurrent illness, hyperemesis, non-compliance, medication errors and failure to adjust diabetic treatment when prescribing medications such as β2-agonists and corticosteroids, which may be given for tocolysis and for fetal lung maturation, respectively [136,138,139].

Management of DKA in pregnancy is the same as for non-pregnant individuals, involving aggressive intravenous hydration, intravenous insulin infusion and close monitoring for fetal distress. Admission to a high-dependency setting capable of monitoring both mother and fetus is essential. Although non-reassuring fetal heart rate tracings are common, most usually resolve quickly with treatment of DKA [140]. However, continuous fetal monitoring is considered prudent in case emergency delivery is required.

Ketonuria may be associated with the development of DKA but is not uncommon in the early-morning urine of non-diabetic women (7%) and has been found in up to 19% of diabetic women limited to a 1,000-calorie daily diet in whom it reflects the effect of overnight starvation [141]. Ketonuria is not necessarily accompanied by serum ketosis and in isolation has not been found to have an adverse effect on the neonate with respect to APGAR scores [141].

Hypoglycaemia

The risk of hypoglycaemia increases as treatment is optimised to meet glycaemic targets. The risk is highest for women with pre-existing diabetes, particularly type 1 diabetics, in whom the rate can be as high as 45% [142,143] especially in the first trimester when insulin therapy is increased to achieve normoglycaemia and there may be hyperemesis. Pre-disposing risk factors include a recent history of severe hypoglycaemia, hypoglycaemia unawareness, longer duration of diabetes, lower HbA1c in early pregnancy, fluctuating blood glucose levels, and excessive use of supplementary insulin between meals [144]. Severe hypoglycaemia during pregnancy can result in maternal mortality [145], but does not appear to increase the risk of congenital malformations, pre-eclampsia, preterm delivery or growth restriction [144]. Women need to be made aware of the increased risk of hypoglycaemia and advised to carry rapidly released sources of glucose or a glucagon pen [146].

Fetal Surveillance and Management

Surveillance

As discussed above, poorly controlled diabetes can have several adverse effects on the fetus. These include increased risk of miscarriages [17], congenital anomalies [147] and growth disorders like macrosomia or fetal growth restriction [148,149]. Fetal risks occurring in early pregnancy primarily affect pregnancies complicated by pre-existing diabetes and much less commonly gestational diabetes, unless it is hitherto undiagnosed and already poorly controlled as indicated by the HbA1c [150].

All women should be offered a first-trimester scan for viability and accurate dating. Diabetes adversely affects performance of the second-trimester maternal serum screening test for fetal chromosomal anomalies, so an early scan allows the option to undergo first-trimester combined screening test using fetal nuchal translucency measurements and maternal biochemistry. An alternative is to use free fetal DNA analysis in a maternal blood sample, but this test remains more expensive than biochemical testing and is not currently as widely available. The main congenital malformations are neural tube defects and congenital cardiac anomalies, which predominate at four times risk of general population [151,152]. The main late pregnancy complications affecting the fetus are growth disorders, such as macrosomia but also fetal growth restriction (FGR), especially in women with pre-existing diabetes with vascular complications, stillbirth and polyhydramnios, which may reflect poor maternal glycaemic control and predispose to preterm labour.

A detailed fetal anomaly scan at 18–22 weeks and fetal echocardiography at 22 weeks should be performed, with serial growth scans throughout pregnancy. The NICE Guidelines advise offering pregnant women with diabetes ultrasound monitoring of fetal growth and amniotic fluid volume every 4 weeks from 28 to 36 weeks [36]. The Guidelines also state that routine monitoring of fetal well-being (using methods such as fetal umbilical artery Doppler recording, fetal heart rate recording and biophysical profile testing) before 38 weeks is not recommended in pregnant women with diabetes unless there is a risk of fetal growth restriction. The Guidelines further suggest providing an individualised approach to monitoring fetal growth and well-being for those women with diabetes and a risk of fetal growth restriction (for example, macrovascular disease or nephropathy).

Macrosomia

The incidence of macrosomia has been reported as between 8% and 43% [148,149] and is mainly explained by fetal hyperinsulinaemia from fetal pancreatic stimulation by fetal hyperglycaemia secondary to maternal hyperglycaemia [153]. There are many definitions of macrosomia, usually related to the given population with norms being derived from standardized populations. It may also be defined in terms of an absolute birth weight of more than 4,000 g or 4,500 g. The pattern of accelerated fetal growth in diabetic pregnancies is characterised by a decreased head-to-abdominal circumference ratio, an increased skinfold thickness and a widened bisacromial diameter, which is responsible for an increased risk of shoulder dystocia at birth at any given birth weight [154,155].

The Hyperglycaemia and Adverse Pregnancy Outcomes (HAPO) study demonstrated that the risk of adverse maternal, fetal, and neonatal outcomes including macrosomia and shoulder dystocia were positively and linearly correlated with maternal glycaemia between 24 and 28 weeks of gestation [79]. There is currently no agreement on the optimum gestational age or the level of maternal hyperglycaemia that predicts the extent of fetal macrosomia. Some have found that postprandial glucose values and/or HbA1c are the best predictors of fetal macrosomia [116,156].

A retrospective series of growth scans in patients with diet-controlled GDM showed that a fetal abdominal circumference measurement above the 90th percentile at 30–33 weeks' gestation had a sensitivity of 88% and a specificity of 83% for he prediction of birth weight >90th percentile [157]. This was better than ultrasound-estimated fetal weights, which include additional head and limb measurements which had poorer sensitivity and positive predictive values for macrosomia.

Fetal Growth Restriction

This is likely to affect pregnancies complicated by pre-existing diabetic women with vascular complications that can affect the placenta. Particular attention needs to be paid to women with poor glycaemic control but who have an apparently normal sized baby. This may indicate a relatively growth-restricted fetus (with normal abdominal circumference) and in this particular situation regular assessment including Doppler studies and cardiotocography (CTG) may be justified. Such fetuses are at particular risk of intrauterine demise and early delivery may be prudent [158].

Neither routine antenatal CTG or Doppler assessment have a clear role in antenatal surveillance of pregnancies complicated by diabetes because of their limited ability to detect sudden fetal compromise, especially in GDM with no other secondary pregnancy complications. However, CTG changes are seen with fetal hypoxia, acidosis and hypoxia, all of which can result from complications of diabetes and require urgent action. There have been case reports of normalisation of the CTG after stabilisation of the mother and correction of the biochemical abnormalities, which raises the possibility of adopting a conservative approach, especially at extremely early gestations. However, once the fetus has reached viability and likely pulmonary maturity, delivery is usually considered the safest option to avoid intrauterine death [140]. Jabak et al. showed that diabetics on insulin were at higher risk of developing a pathological CTG and therefore benefit from continuous intrapartum monitoring [159].

Doppler assessment does appear to have a role in pregnancies in diabetic women with vasculopathy who are at a higher risk of having a fetus with growth restriction. Pietryga et al., in a retrospective study of 155 women with pregestational diabetes between 22 and 40 weeks, found that abnormal umbilical waveforms and uterine notching were related to maternal vasculopathy, as indicated by the White classification and associated with poor pregnancy outcomes, suggesting the vasculopathy also affects the uterine arteries potentially influencing placental perfusion and fetal well-being [160].

Preterm Labour

A cohort study of more than 46,000 pregnancies excluding women with pre-existing diabetes showed a direct relationship (RR 1.42; 95% CI 1.15 to 1.77) between the risk of spontaneous preterm delivery and maternal blood glucose, independent of other factors associated with prematurity [131]. Spontaneous preterm birth among the women with GDM was increased when the mean blood glucose was >5.8 mmol/l (OR 1.94, 95% CI 1.25 to 3.0) [156].

Tocolytics

Atosiban, an oxytocin receptor antagonist, and nifedipine, a calcium channel blocker, can be used in diabetics in cases of threatened or actual preterm labour. Howeveer, β_2-adrenergic agonists such as salbutamol and ritodrine may worsen maternal hyperglycaemia and should be avoided [161].

Corticosteroids

Prenatal corticosteroids should be given for obstetric indications and not avoided because of their potential for increasing maternal blood glucose levels. Women in whom antenatal corticosteroids are indicated may require hospitalisation for closer monitoring of the blood glucose levels in anticipation of the likely need for increased insulin doses. In one study of corticosteroids given to mothers with type 1 diabetes, it was noted that the insulin requirement increased by 20% on days 1 and 4, by 40% on days 2 and 3, and returned to the pre-existing dose on days 6 and 7 [162]. Late administration of corticosteroids beyond 34 weeks is no longer recommended and should probably be avoided because of the resultant maternal hyperglycaemia in diabetic mothers and even diabetic ketoacidosis in patients with GDM [163], although randomised trials of such administration at 33–36 weeks are currently being performed (www.ligginstrials.org/Precede_Test/) [164], and recommendations may change as a result.

Management Options – Labour and Delivery

Timing and Mode of Delivery

A delivery plan for pregnant women with diabetes is influenced by:

- The degree of glycaemic control during the pregnancy
- Whether maternal complications are present (e.g., hypertension, pre-eclampsia, worsening retinopathy or nephropathy)
- The woman's past obstetric history
- The gestational age (concern about the risk of stillbirth often underpins a decision for an elective delivery before the estimated date of delivery)
- Whether there is pathological fetal growth (e.g. macrosomia, growth restriction)

Recommendations for the timing and mode of delivery differ between those with pre-existing diabetes and GDM. In cases of well-controlled GDM without fetal complications the absolute risk of stillbirth and infant death is low and the risks of expectant management are similar to a non-diabetic pregnancy [165]. Thus, the NICE guidelines recommend that for women with diet-controlled GDM with no other risk factors, delivery should occur no later than 40^{+6} weeks by induction of labour, or obstetrically indicated Caesarean section [42].

The timing and mode of delivery for women with pre-existing DM on insulin should be individualised and involve a multidisciplinary discussion between the medical team including obstetrician, obstetric physician or endocrinologist and anaesthetist and the woman. In specific cases, involvement of a neonatal paediatrician may necessary.

For pregnant women with pre-existing diabetes with a normally grown fetus, the NICE guideline recommends that elective birth by induction of labour, or elective Caesarean section if indicated, should be offered after 38 completed weeks [42]. Boulvain et al. showed that induction of labour between 37 and 39 weeks for suspected fetal macrosomia was associated with higher rates of vaginal birth (RR 1.14, 95% CI 1.01 to 1.29) and a reduction in the shoulder dystocia rate (RR 0.32, 95% CI 0.12 to 0.85) [166] when compared to women awaiting spontaneous onset of labour. Elective Caesarean section should be considered for any woman with diabetes if the estimated fetal weight is greater than 4.5 kg [42].

Pregnant women need to be advised about the risks of birth injury including shoulder dystocia, especially for a macrosomic fetus. Studies have suggested a 0.58–0.70% incidence of shoulder dystocia in non-diabetic women and the risk for an infant of a diabetic mother is between two and four times that of a non-diabetic at the same gestational weight [126,167]. Following a sentinel medicolegal case in the UK (*Montgomery versus Lanarkshire*), advising diabetic pregnant women of the risk of shoulder dystocia has been strongly recommended with the offer of an alternative option of a Caesarean delivery where there is suspected fetal macrosomia [168].

The decision on timing of delivery should be individualised and take into consideration the type of DM, the degree of glycaemic control and whether there are fetal complications. The main aim of early delivery in those with pre-existing diabetes is stillbirth prevention. The recommendation of delivery between 37 and 38 completed weeks' gestation if the glycaemic control is good reflects the balance of risks between that of respiratory distress (both respiratory distress syndrome (RDS) and transient tachypnoea (TTN)) due to earlier delivery and that of fetal demise if the pregnancy is allowed to continue [93]. Despite an upper limit for delivery of 38 weeks for diabetic mothers in general, with poorly controlled diabetes or fetal macrosomia, it is recommended that delivery can be offered even before 37 weeks to reduce the risk of unexpected fetal demise and birth injuries from instrumental vaginal deliveries associated with fetal macrosomia [169].

Maternal obesity, which itself is often linked with type 2 diabetes and a risk factor for GDM, has been associated with an increased risk of perinatal death. The risk of asphyxia and perinatal death is also increased in infants with severe macrosomia regardless of the cause of macrosomia [170].

Management of Labour

Delivery of a diabetic mother should take place in a facility with 24-hour anaesthetic cover, a neonatal unit and staff with expertise to care for women with DM and their babies. The NICE suggests that all diabetic women in active labour should have continuous electronic fetal monitoring [42].

Peripartum Glycaemic Management

The main goal of good peripartum glycaemic control is to minimise the incidence of neonatal hypoglycaemia, thought to be due to fetal hyperinsulinism induced by maternal hyperglycaemia. The target peripartum blood glucose level is between 4 and 7 mmol/l [30,76]. This is usually achieved by means of an intravenous insulin infusion and dextrose drip, with hourly capillary blood glucose monitoring and infusion rate adjustments using a sliding scale [171]. Women receiving insulin pump therapy can continue to use their insulin pump in labour with similar adjustments on the basis of the glucose monitoring. They usually require suspension of the basal insulin during active labour and resumption of their pre-pregnancy pump settings postpartum.

First Stage of Labour

In the latent phase of labour diabetic women should be allowed a normal diet and encouraged to ambulate. During the active phase, the mother has lower insulin requirements because increased calorie consumption and reduced calorific intake lead to a small fall in her blood glucose level. Theoretically, this can result in the fetus also being exposed to low glucose levels (glucose passes readily across the placenta by facilitated diffusion via hexose transporters that are not dependent on maternal insulin but are regulated only by the maternal–fetal concentration gradient, so fetal blood glucose levels are signficantly correlated with maternal values), making it less able to cope with the intermittent hypoxia produced by contractions.

Second Stage of Labour

The risk of shoulder dystocia is highest when there is a combination of fetal macrosomia, prolonged labour and a mid-cavity instrumental delivery, especially by vacuum. The decision for such a delivery needs to be made by a senior obstetrician and should be considered a 'trial of instrumental delivery' and preferably performed in the operating theatre [155] with early recourse to Caesarean section, if unsuccessful.

Anesthesia and Analegesia

The obstetric anaesthetist is a key member of the multidisciplinary team and, as stated above, needs to be aware of any diabetic patient in labour. The NICE Guidelines recommend an anaesthetic assessment in the third trimester for all women with complicated diabetes [42]. If general anaesthesia is used, the blood glucose level should be monitored regularly from induction of general anaesthesia until the woman is fully conscious. For intravenous pre-hydration before operative anaesthesia, a normal saline-containing crystalloid is usually used rather than a dextrose-containing solution, to avoid administering a large glucose load, which can lead to neonatal hypoglycaemia [172].

Management Options – Postnatal

Maternal Care

Following delivery, maternal glycaemic control returns rapidly to that seen before the pregnancy and needs to be actively managed in the immediate postpartum period to avoid glycaemic instability. Management differs between women with pre-existing diabetes who may or may not need to continue insulin and true gestational diabetic women who become normoglycaemic after birth and can discontinue medication.

a. Pharmacotherapy for Pre-existing Diabetes

Women with T1DM may generally resume their pre-pregnancy insulin regimens. Women with T2DM may continue metformin therapy, as it is excreted only minimally in breast milk. Breastfeeding lowers blood glucose levels and lactating mothers may require further insulin dose reductions, or a carbohydrate snack prior to breastfeeding to avoid hypoglycaemia. Glyburide and glipizide are undetectable in breast milk, and may also be used during breastfeeding [173]. Limited information is available for other sulphonylureas and GLP-1 receptor analogues and are therefore not recommended during lactation and insulin may be required if the blood sugar level remains high.

About 90% of women with GDM return to normal glucose tolerance immediately after delivery [70] and therefore glucose-lowering treatment should then be discontinued. Recommendations for screening following a pregnancy affected by GDM varies around the globe, but most professional societies recommend one postpartum OGTT at 6–12 weeks to detect those with previously undiagnosed hyperglycaemia followed by annual screening. It is recommended by NICE that all women with GDM should be offered a 75-g, 2-hour OGTT at 4–12 weeks postpartum, and repeat testing every 1–3 years thereafter if this is normal, to detect women who have or who develop T2DM. Alternatively, women diagnosed with GDM with negative postpartum testing for diabetes can be offered annual HbA1c testing [39].

The risk of progression to type 2 diabetes following a pregnancy complicated by GDM varies between 15% and 50% at 5 years [4,174]. These women should be given lifestyle advice regarding diet, exercise and weight management to decrease, or at least delay, their risk of developing type 2 diabetes later in life [4].

b. Lactation

Women should be educated about the benefits of breastfeeding for the baby and their own metabolic health [174]. Medications prescribed should be safe for breastfeeding.

c. Contraception

Contraception advice is a vital yet often overlooked component of postpartum care. This should be individualised and discussed postnatally before discharge, especially if the patient is at risk of defaulting her postnatal visits. Important considerations for choice of appropriate contraceptive include the presence of diabetic complications, breastfeeding, smoking, age and plans for future fertility. The WHO guidelines on contraceptive use can be used (see Table 7) [175].

Neonatal Care

Babies of mothers with diabetes are at increased risk of morbidity and mortality compared with neonates born to mothers without diabetes and need a detailed postnatal examination. Management of the neonate requires anticipation of the possible complications associated with exposure to maternal hyperglycaemia. These include [177]:

- metabolic complications (hypoglycaemia, hypocalcaemia, and hypomagnesaemia)
- hematologic complications (polycythaemia and hyperviscosity)
- hyperbilirubinaemia
- fetal cardiomegaly

Table 7 WHO contraception guidelines in diabetes mellitus [176]

Condition	CHC	POP	DMPA/ NET-EN	IMP	Cu IUD	IUS
History of gestational diabetes	I	I	I	I	I	I
Non-vascular disease						
i. Non-insulin-dependent	2	2	2	2	I	2
ii. Insulin-dependent	2	2	2	2	I	2
Neuropathy/retinopathy/neuropathy	3/4	2	3	2	I	2
Other vascular disease	3/4	2	3	2	I	2

Abbreviations: CHC, combined hormonal contraception; Cu IUD, copper intrauterine device; DMPA/NET-EN, medroxyprogesterone acetate/Norethisterone enanthate; IMP, implants; POP, progestogen-only pill; IUS, intrauterine system.
Key: 1, no restriction for the use of the contraceptive method; 2, advantages of using the method generally outweigh the theoretical or proven risks; 3, theoretical or proven risks usually outweigh the advantages of the method; 4, unacceptable health risk if the contraceptive method is used.

Neonatal Hypoglycaemia

Neonatal hypoglycaemia (plasma glucose < 2 mmol/l) is caused by the persistence of fetal hyperinsulinaemia after birth, especially when maternal glycaemia has been poorly controlled in pregnancy. Insulin inhibits the activation of metabolic pathways of glucose production that normally occur in healthy newborns and increases glucose consumption by the tissues. Maternal hyperglycaemia during labour can stimulate excessive secretion of fetal insulin for 1–2 hours after birth and cause neonatal hypoglycaemia [170].

Neonates of mothers with diabetes should be fed as soon as possible after delivery (within 30 minutes) and then at frequent intervals (every 2–3 hours) until prefeed capillary plasma glucose is maintained at a minimum of 2.0 mmol/l [42]. Blood glucose testing should be carried out 2–4 hours after birth or if the baby exhibit symptoms and/or signs consistent with hypoglycaemia. The rate of neonatal hypoglycaemia requiring intravenous glucose therapy among babies of GDM mothers is low (<5%) in several studies. Long-term outcome data have suggested that prenatal exposure to hyperglycaemia increases the risk of postnatal metabolic complications including type 2 diabetes and obesity [178,179].

Hypocalcaemia and Hyperbilirubinaemia

Babies born to women with pre-existing diabetes have an increased risk of neonatal hypocalcaemia of between 20% and 60% [180,181]. In contrast, babies born to women with GDM have a very low risk (<1%). In the presence of symptoms compatible with hypocalcaemia or hypomagnesaemia (e.g. jitteriness or seizure), serum calcium and magnesium levels should be measured. If there is clinical suspicion of jaundice, serum bilirubin level should be checked. The risk of hyperbilirubinaemia in babies of GDM mothers (after making allowance for preterm delivery) has not been found to be markedly increased [170].

Polycythaemia

Polycythaemia (venous haematocrit ≥65%) is more common in infants of diabetic mothers. It is thought possibly to be due to elevated erythropoietin levels from chronic intrauterine hypoxia. It has also been associated with hypocalcaemia and hypomagnesaemia in these infants although there is no direct relationship between calcium and magnesium levels and the hematocrit [182]. Measurement of hematocrit should be performed within the first few hours of birth to exclude polycythaemia.

Fetal Cardiomegaly

Myocardial hypertrophy has been reported in fetuses and newborns of mothers with diabetes [170]. This is characterised by myofibrillar hypertrophy and hyperplasia, without myocardial fiber disarray [183]. This leads to hypertrophy of the ventricular walls, predominantly involving the septum. The pathophysiology of fetal cardiomyopathy is unknown but may be linked to fetal hyperinsulinaemia. Myocardial hypertrophy is associated with decreased ventricular compliance and increased contractility of both ventricles. In its most advanced form, major septal hypertrophy can lead to subaortic stenosis and secondary mitral insufficiency. An echocardiogram is indicated if the baby demonstrates clinical signs (including cardiac murmur) associated with congenital heart disease or cardiomyopathy [36].

Long-term Risks Following a Pregnancy Affected by GDM

A diagnosis of GDM has future implications for both the mother and her baby. The most notable risk for the mother, perhaps, is the development of type 2 diabetes, but GDM is also associated with a threefold future risk of metabolic syndrome (obesity, hypertension, insulin resistance and dyslipidaemia), cardiovascular disease and death due to vascular endothelial dysfunction [184]. It has been linked with the subsequent development of ophthalmic and renal disease and malignancies [185,186].

Women diagnosed with GDM with an abnormal postnatal OGTT should be referred for long-term outpatient management of their impaired glucose tolerance. Women with a normal postnatal OGTT can be reassured, but do need to be advised of their increased risk of developing future T2DM and the need for annual testing to prevent the development of large vessel and microvascular complications of undiagnosed disease. The importance of maintaining a healthy lifestyle in terms of diet and exercise, which clinical trials have suggested can reduce the risk or at least delay the onset of T2DM, should be stressed [187].

The children of mothers diagnosed with GDM are also at up to eight times the risk of developing prediabetes and diabetes as adolescents as well as obesity in comparison to children of non-diabetic mothers, thus perpetuating the cycle [184]. They are also more prone to other endocrine disorders and hypertension [185]. These effects have been linked with fetal nutritional status. The developmental origins of health and disease hypothesis proposes that in-utero undernourishment leads the child to develop diabetes and hypertension in future life if it receives adequate nutrition after birth. Children of mothers who had GDM are also at risk of paediatric ophthalmic morbidities, impaired neurodevelopmental outcome and long-term neuropsychiatric morbidities including autism and eating disorders [188,189].

7 Summary of Management Options for Diabetes in Pregnancy

Pre-pregnancy

Overall care by multidisciplinary team involving the woman in management decisions

Pre-pregnancy counselling:
- Risks of pregnancy
- Importance of good blood glucose control and options for treatment
- Use of effective contraception until good glycaemic control
- Folate supplementation (5 mg daily)
- Prompt contact once pregnant

Glycaemic targets:
- HbA1c ≤ 6.5 if safely achievable
- Advise to avoid conception if HbA1c ≥ 10%

Self-monitoring of blood glucose and blood ketones:
- Aim for non-diabetic pre- and postprandial glucose values – see Table 2 for values from different Guidelines
- Test for ketonaemia if hyperglycaemic or unwell

Diet and body weight:
- Take folic acid 5 mg daily until 12 weeks' gestation
- Offer nutritional and exercise advice: obese women should try and reduce their weight

(cont.)

Glucose-lowering drugs:
- Metformin would appear to be safe in the first trimester so can be taken pre-pregnancy; the safety of other oral hypoglycaemic agents is not as well documented, although glibenclimide has been considered safe by one Guideline. If the patient is on other oral agents, a change to metformin or insulin is recommended
- Women taking split-dose premixed insulin should switch to multiple single-agent injections to optimise glycaemic control
- If good glycaemic control with insulin glargine then it is probably safe to continue
- Hybrid closed-loop insulin therapy has been shown to be very effective in management of women with type 1 disease

Management of comorbid conditions:
- Hypertension: aim to keep blood pressure (BP) < 130/85 mmHg; change from ACE inhibitors or ARBs to methyldopa or labetalol, which have a safer pregnancy track record; avoid BP >120/80 mmHg
- Dyslipidaemia: discontinue statins, fibrates and niacin; offer dietary counselling with hypertriglyceridaemia
- Thyroid disease: assess TSH in women with T1DM and measure thyroid peroxidase antibodies

Management of diabetes-related conditions:
- Retinopathy: ophthalmic review and treatment if necessary
- Nephropathy: assess renal function; careful counselling about risks of pregnancy for women with severe nephropathy (raised creatinine and decreased GFR); review of drugs and risks for pregnancy
- Repeat ophthalmic and/or renal assessment if not undertaken within 6 months of a pregnancy
- Cardiovascular disease: women with a history of ischaemic heart disease should be offered a cardiological review before considering conception; careful counselling about risks of conceiving in these cases

Prenatal

Offer antenatal care through a multidisciplinary clinic:
- See Table 6 for a suggested maternal and fetal surveillance programme

GDM – screening and diagnosis (see Table 3):
- Options for screening: there are differences in published guidelines about the method used (total population/'universal' screening or only women with risk factors) and the screening method

(cont.)

- Options for diagnosis: this is by an OGTT and there is greater consistency between the guidelines about the criteria for diagnosis

GDM – specific interventions once diagnosed:

- Education about management of pregnancy and minimising the risks
- Teach SMBG (same targets as for women with pre-existing diabetes – see Table 4)
- Dietary referral and advice
- Possible therapeutic strategy:
  - Start metformin if fasting plasma glucose < 7 mmol/l
  - Start or add insulin if fasting plasma glucose ≥ 7 mmol/l or poor control on diet, exercise and metformin

Blood glucose monitoring:

- Frequency: recommendations vary, but commonly at least 7 times daily (fasting, pre- and 1 hour post-meals) with pregestational diabetes and multiple insulin injections; 4 times daily (post-meals) with diet/oral/long-acting insulin
- Targets:
  - See Table 4

Ketone monitoring:

- Women with type 1 diabetes should measure their blood ketone levels if they are hyperglycaemic or unwell
- If ketonaemic, the woman should seek urgent medical assistance
- Women with type 2 diabetes or GDM need not routinely check their ketone levels

Diet and exercise:

- Targeted calorie-controlled low glycaemic index diet
- Moderate exercise (such as walking after meals for 30 minutes) daily

Treatment:

- Oral hypoglycaemic agents
  - Metformin will achieve glycaemic control in most women with type 2 diabetes and GDM
  - Glyburide can be used if women do not attain glucose targets on optimal metformin dose and decline insulin treatment, or if they are intolerant of metformin
- Insulin
  - Most insulins have a good safety record in pregnancy; the main exception is insulin glulisine
  - Use a multidose regimen (e.g. 4 times daily) and titrate insulin dose according to the fasting, pre- and postprandial glucose values

(cont.)

Maternal surveillance and management of complications:
- Retinopathy: examine retinae each trimester and for one year postpartum; pan-retinal laser coagulation can be used in pregnancy; use of anti-VEGF medications needs a risk–benefit discussion with the woman
- Nephropathy: assess basal renal function at the beginning of the pregnancy and repeat if abnormal
- Hypertension: aim to keep BP between 120/80 and 135/85 mmHg
- Hypoglycaemia: the woman needs to remain vigilant and carry rapidly released sources of glucose and/or a glucagon pen

Diabetic ketoacidosis (DKA):
- Maintain vigilance for this complication in all pregnant women with diabetes
- Manage DKA as in a non-pregnant patient (volume replacement, IV insulin, correct electrolyte disturbance and address precipitating cause)
- DKA is not an indication for delivery
- Intermittent ketonuria (especially in early-morning specimens) is not uncommon
- Persistent ketonuria is an indication for testing for serum ketosis; if that is confirmed, manage as DKA

Fetal surveillance:
- Accurate ultrasound dating in first trimester
- Offer Down syndrome screening
- Detailed fetal anomaly scan at about 20 weeks and further fetal cardiac scan at 22 weeks
- Check fetal growth and amniotic fluid volume at 28, 32 and 36 weeks (abdominal circumference and/or head abdomen ratio are the most accurate predictors of macrosomia)
- Routine monitoring of fetal well-being (including fetal umbilical artery Doppler recording, fetal heart rate recording and biophysical profile testing) before 38 weeks is not recommended in pregnant women with diabetes, unless there is a risk of fetal growth restriction
- Provide an individualised approach to monitoring fetal growth and well-being for women with diabetes and a risk of fetal growth restriction (for example, macrovascular disease or nephropathy)
- There is insufficient evidence to recommend using ultrasound assessment of fetal size to determine insulin treatment

Preterm labour and delivery:
- Risk is greater with poor glycaemic control
- Calcium channel blockers and oxytocin receptor antagonists can be used; avoid β_2-adrenergic agonists

(cont.)

- Corticosteroids should be used for the normal indications, but increased insulin doses will be needed to cover the resultant temporary hyperglycaemia

---

Labour and delivery

Timing and mode of birth:
- Influenced by glycaemic control, maternal complications, past obstetric history, gestational age, pathological fetal growth (macrosomia or growth restriction)
- Offer elective delivery at 37^{+0}–38^{+6} weeks in women with pre-existing diabetes
- Offer elective delivery at no later than 40^{+6} weeks in women with GDM with no complications and whose diabetes is well controlled
- Discuss the potential for shoulder dystocia with women before labour; consider elective Caesarean section if estimated fetal weight $\geq$ 4,500 g

Delivery should take place in centres with 24-hour anaesthetic cover, a neonatal intensive care unit and staff trained in the care of women with diabetes

Use protocols for care in labour covering:
- Blood glucose control
  - Capillary glucose values every 4 hours (more frequently if poor control)
  - Aim for 4.0–7.0 mmol/l
- Woman can be mobile, and can eat and drink normally, in early labour
- A dextrose/insulin infusion will be necessary in many diabetic labours
- Continuous fetal heart rate monitoring
- Vigilance for shoulder dystocia in second stage
- Consider anaesthetic consultation in third trimester of pregnancy for obese women and those with autonomic neuropathy

---

Postnatal/neonatal

Change medical management immediately after delivery:
- Return women with pre-existing diabetes to their pre-pregnancy insulin/hypoglycaemic therapy
- Discontinue hypoglycaemic therapy in women with GDM, and monitor blood glucose levels for evidence of newly diagnosed type 2 diabetes

Women with GDM:
- Give advice about diet, exercise and weight management
- Inform about risk of recurrence of GDM in future pregnancy

(cont.)

- Offer 75-g OGTT at 6 weeks postnatal
- Advise annual 75-g OGTT

Encourage breastfeeding; metformin and glyburide are safe for breastfeeding
Offer contraceptive advice

Newborn:
- Early feeding and monitor capillary glucose values; most babies can be managed with extra feeding and not IV dextrose
- Screen/surveillance for metabolic complications, haematological complications, hyperbilirubinaemia, cardiomegaly, congenital abnormality

ACE, angiotensin-converting enzyme; ARB, angiotensin receptor blocker; BP, blood pressure; DKA, diabetic ketoacidosis; FGR, fetal growth restriction; GDM, gestational diabetes mellitus; GFR, glomerular filtration rate; HbA1c, hemoglobin A1c; IV, intravenous; OGTT, oral glucose tolerance test; SMBG, self-monitoring of blood glucose.

Key References

Australia

Rudland VL, Price SAL, Hughes R, et al. ADIPS 2020 guideline for pre-existing diabetes and pregnancy. *Aust N Z J Obstet Gynaecol*. 2020 Dec;60(6):E18–E52. https://doi.org/10.1111/ajo.13265. Epub 2020 Nov 16. PMID: 33200400.

Shub A. Diabetes and pregnancy. *Aust N Z J Obstet Gynaecol*. 2020; 60: 829–30. doi: 10.1111/ajo.13275. PMID: 33373054.

FIGO

Hod M, Kapur A, Sacks DA, et al. The International Federation of Gynecology and Obstetrics (FIGO) Initiative on gestational diabetes mellitus: A pragmatic guide for diagnosis, management, and care. *Int J Gynaecol Obstet*. 2015 Oct;131(Suppl 3): S173–211. https://doi.org/10.1016/S0020-7292(15)30033-3. PMID: 26433807.

Canada

Berger H, Gagnon R, Sermer M. Guideline No. 393 – Diabetes in Pregnancy. *J Obstet Gynaecol Can*. 2019;4:1814–25.e1. https://doi.org/10.1016/j.jogc .2019.03.008. Erratum in: *J Obstet Gynaecol Can*. 2020 Oct; 42:1288. PMID: 31785800.

Diabetes Canada Clinical Practice Guidelines Expert Committee; Feig DS, Berger H, et al. Diabetes and pregnancy. *Can J Diabetes*. 2018 Apr;42(Suppl 1): S255–82. https://doi.org/10.1016/j.jcjd.2017.10.038. Erratum in: *Can J Diabetes*. 2018 Jun;42(3):337. PMID: 29650105.

Sweden

Goldberg A, Ursing C, Ekéus C, Wiberg-Itzel E. Swedish guidelines for type 1 diabetes and pregnancy outcomes: A nationwide descriptive study of consensus and adherence. *Prim Care Diabetes*. 2021;15:1040–51. https://doi.org/10.1016/ j.pcd.2021.08.003. Epub 2021 Sep 21. PMID: 34556439.

USA

ACOG Guidance on Perinatal Management of Pregestational Diabetes [cited 2023 Mar 14]. www.obgproject.com/2018/12/18/updated-acog-guidance-on-perinatal-management-of-pregestational-diabetes/.

ACOG Practice Bulletin No. 190 Summary: Gestational Diabetes Mellitus. *Obstet Gynecol*. 2018 Feb;131(2):406–08. https://doi.org/10.1097/ AOG.0000000000002498. PMID: 29370044.

American Diabetes Association. 14. Management of Diabetes in Pregnancy & Standards of Medical Care in Diabetes – 2020. *Diabetes Care*. 2020 Jan;43 (Suppl 1):S183–92. https://doi.org/10.2337/dc20-S014. PMID: 31862757.

UK

NICE Diabetes in Pregnancy: Management of diabetes and its complications from pre-conception to the postnatal period (accessed 1/3/23). www.nice.org .uk/Guidance/NG3.

NICE Diabetes in pregnancy: Quality Standard (QS109) (accessed 1/3/23). www.nice.org.uk/guidance/qs109.

Reviews

Crowther CA, Samuel D, Hughes R, et al. ; TARGET Study Group. Tighter or less tight glycaemic targets for women with gestational diabetes mellitus for reducing maternal and perinatal morbidity: A stepped-wedge, cluster-randomised trial. *PLoS Med*. 2022 Sep 8;19(9):e1004087. https://doi.org/10.1371/journal .pmed.1004087. PMID: 36074760; PMCID: PMC9455881.

ElSayed NA, Aleppo G, Aroda VR, et al., on behalf of the American Diabetes Association. 2. Classification and Diagnosis of Diabetes: Standards of Care in Diabetes – 2023. *Diabetes Care*. 2023 Jan 1;46(Suppl 1):S19–40. https://doi .org/10.2337/dc23-S002. Erratum in: *Diabetes Care*. 2023 Feb 01: PMID: 36507649; PMCID: PMC9810477.

Gemmill A, Leonard SA. Risk of adverse pregnancy outcomes among US individuals with gestational diabetes by race and ethnicity. *JAMA*. 2022 Jul 26;328(4):397. https://doi.org/10.1001/jama.2022.9412. PMID: 35881129.

Murphy HR, Howgate C, O'Keefe J, et al.; National Pregnancy in Diabetes (NPID) advisory group. Characteristics and outcomes of pregnant women with type 1 or type 2 diabetes: A 5-year national population-based cohort study. *Lancet Diabetes Endocrinol*. 2021;9:153–64. https://doi.org/10.1016/S2213-8587(20)30406-X. Epub 2021 Jan 28. PMID: 33516295.

Relph S, Patel T, Delaney L, Sobhy S, Thangaratinam S. Adverse pregnancy outcomes in women with diabetes-related microvascular disease and risks of disease progression in pregnancy: A systematic review and meta-analysis. *PLoS Med*. 2021 Nov 22;18(11):e1003856. https://doi.org/10.1371/journal .pmed.1003856. PMID: 34807920; PMCID: PMC8654151.

Ye W, Luo C, Huang J, et al. Gestational diabetes mellitus and adverse pregnancy outcomes: Systematic review and meta-analysis. *BMJ*. 2022 May 25;377:e067946. https://doi.org/10.1136/bmj-2021-067946. PMID: 35613728; PMCID: PMC9131781.

Full References

1. Relph S, Patel T, Delaney L, Sobhy S, Thangaratinam S. Adverse pregnancy outcomes in women with diabetes-related microvascular disease and risks of disease progression in pregnancy: A systematic review and meta-analysis. *PLoS Med.* 2021 Nov;18(11):e1003856.

2. Ye W, Luo C, Huang J, et al. Gestational diabetes mellitus and adverse pregnancy outcomes: Systematic review and meta-analysis. *BMJ.* 2022 May 25;377:e067946.

3. Hannah W, Bhavadharini B, Beks H, et al. Global burden of early pregnancy gestational diabetes mellitus (eGDM): A systematic review. *Acta Diabetol.* 2022 Mar;59(3):403–27.

4. Sweeting A, Wong J, Murphy HR, Ross GP. A clinical update on gestational diabetes mellitus. *Endocr Rev.* 2022 Sep 26;43(5):763–93.

5. Peng TY, Ehrlich SF, Crites Y, et al. Trends and racial and ethnic disparities in the prevalence of pregestational type 1 and type 2 diabetes in Northern California: 1996–2014. *Am J Obstet Gynecol.* 2017 Feb;216(2):177.e1–177.e8.

6. Jovanovič L, Liang Y, Weng W, et al. Trends in the incidence of diabetes, its clinical sequelae, and associated costs in pregnancy. *Diabetes Metab Res Rev.* 2015 Oct;31(7):707–16.

7. Egan AM, Dunne FP. Epidemiology of gestational and pregestational diabetes mellitus. In: Lapolla A, Metzger BE, editors. *Frontiers in Diabetes* [Internet]. S. Karger AG; 2020 [cited 2023 Feb 25]. pp. 1–10. www.karger.com/Article/FullText/480161.

8. Lam AYR, Lim W, McMicking J, et al. *The Global Library of Women's Medicine.* www.glowm.com/article/heading/vol-8–maternal-medical-health-and-disorders-in-pregnancy–clinical-management-of-diabetes-in-pregnancy/id/416423

9. Freinkel N. Banting Lecture 1980: Of pregnancy and progeny. *Diabetes.* 1980;29(12):1023–35.

10. Bellamy L, Casas J-P, Hingorani AD, et al. Type 2 diabetes mellitus after gestational diabetes: A systematic review and meta-analysis. *Lancet.* 2009;373(9677):1773–79.

11. Expert Committee on the Diagnosis and Classification of Diabetes Mellitus. Report of the expert committee on the diagnosis and classification of diabetes mellitus. *Diabetes Care.* 2003 Jan; 26(Suppl 1):S5–20.

12. Definition and diagnosis of diabetes mellitus and intermediate hyperglycaemia: Report of a WHO/IDF consultation. Geneva, Switzerland: World Health Organization; 2006.

13. International Expert Committee. International Expert Committee report on the role of the A1 C assay in the diagnosis of diabetes. *Diabetes Care*. 2009 Jul;32(7):1327–34.

14. Faselis C, Katsimardou A, Imprialos K, Deligkaris M, Kallistratos M, Dimitriadis K. Microvascular complications of type 2 diabetes mellitus. *Curr Vasc Pharmacol*. 2020;18(2):117–24.

15. Leguizamón G, Trigubo D, Pereira JI, Vera MF, Fernández JA. Vascular complications in the diabetic pregnancy. *Curr Diab Rep*. 2015 Apr;15 (4):22.

16. Damm JA, Asbjörnsdóttir B, Callesen NF, et al. Diabetic nephropathy and microalbuminuria in pregnant women with type 1 and type 2 diabetes: Prevalence, antihypertensive strategy, and pregnancy outcome. *Diabetes Care*. 2013 Nov;36(11):3489–94.

17. Balsells M, García-Patterson A, Gich I, et al. Major congenital malformations in women with gestational diabetes mellitus: A systematic review and meta-analysis. *Diabetes Metab Res Rev*. 2012;28(3):252–57.

18. Tinker SC, Gilboa SM, Moore CA, et al. Specific birth defects in pregnancies of women with diabetes: National Birth Defects Prevention Study, 1997–2011. *Am J Obstet Gynecol*. 2020 Feb;222(2):176.e1–176.e11.

19. Miodovnik M, Skillman C, Holroyde JC, et al. Elevated maternal glycohemoglobin in early pregnancy and spontaneous abortion among insulin-dependent diabetic women. *Am J Obstet Gynecol*. 1985;153(4):439–42.

20. Temple R, Aldridge V, Greenwood R, et al. Association between outcome of pregnancy and glycemic control in early pregnancy in type 1 diabetes: Population based study. *BMJ*. 2002;325(7375):1275–76.

21. Herman WH, Janz NK, Becker MP, et al. Diabetes and pregnancy. Preconception care, pregnancy outcomes, resource utilization and costs. *J Reprod Med*. 1999;44(1):33–38.

22. Gemmill A, Leonard SA. Risk of adverse pregnancy outcomes among US individuals with gestational diabetes by race and ethnicity. *JAMA*. 2022 Jul 26;328(4):397.

23. Cundy T, Gamble G, Neale L, et al. Differing causes of pregnancy loss in type 1 and type 2 diabetes. *Diabetes Care*. 2007 Oct;30(10):2603–07.

24. Egerup P, Mikkelsen AP, Kolte AM, et al. Pregnancy loss is associated with type 2 diabetes: A nationwide case-control study. *Diabetologia*. 2020 Aug;63(8):1521–29. https://doi.org/10.1007/s00125-020-05154-z.

25. García-Patterson A, Gich I, Amini SB, et al. Insulin requirements throughout pregnancy in women with type 1 diabetes mellitus: Three changes of direction. *Diabetologia*. 2010;53(3):446–51.

26. National Pregnancy in Diabetes (NPID) Audit Report 2020 (accessed 1/3/23). https://files.digital.nhs.uk/4D/0ABE7F/National%20Pregnancy%20in%20Diabetes%20Audit%202020%20Report.pdf.

27. Yamamoto JM, Hughes DJF, Evans ML, et al. Community-based prepregnancy care programme improves pregnancy preparation in women with pregestational diabetes. *Diabetologia*. 2018;61(7):1528–37.

28. Murphy HR, Roland JM, Skinner TC, et al. Effectiveness of a regional prepregnancy care program in women with type 1 and type 2 diabetes: Benefits beyond glycemic control. *Diabetes Care*. 2010;33(12):2514–20.

29. Egan AM, Danyliv A, Carmody L, et al. A prepregnancy care program for women with diabetes: Effective and cost saving. *J Clin Endocrinol Metab*. 2016;101(4):1807–15.

30. American Diabetes Association. 14. Management of Diabetes in Pregnancy: Standards of Medical Care in Diabetes – 2020. *Diabetes Care*. 2020 Jan;43 (Suppl 1):S183–92.

31. Bell R, Glinianaia SV, Tennant PWG, et al. Peri-conception hyperglycaemia and nephropathy are associated with risk of congenital anomaly in women with pre-existing diabetes: A population-based cohort study. *Diabetologia*. 2012; https://doi.org/10.1007/s00125-012-2455-y.

32. Jensen DM, Korsholm L, Ovesen P, et al. Peri-conceptional A1 C and risk of serious adverse pregnancy outcome in 933 women with type 1 diabetes. *Diabetes Care*. 2009;32(6):1046–48.

33. Mills JL, Baker L, Goldman AS. Malformations in infants of diabetic mothers occur before the seventh gestational week. Implications for treatment. *Diabetes*. 1979;28(4):292–93.

34. Nielsen GL, Møller M, Sørensen HT. HbA1c in early diabetic pregnancy and pregnancy outcomes: A Danish population-based cohort study of 573 pregnancies in women with type 1 diabetes. *Diabetes Care*. 2006;29(12):-2612–16.

35. Diabetes Canada Clinical Practice Guidelines Expert Committee, Feig DS, Berger H, et al. Diabetes and pregnancy. *Can J Diabetes*. 2018 Apr;42 (Suppl 1):S255–82.

36. National Collaborating Centre for Women's and Children's Health. Diabetes in pregnancy: Management of diabetes and its complications from preconception to the postnatal period. February 2015. www.nice.org.uk/guidance/ng3.

37. Blumer I, Hadar E, Hadden DR, et al. Diabetes and pregnancy: An endocrine society clinical practice guideline. *J Clin Endocrinol Metab.* 2013;98 (11):4227–49.

38. Feig DS, Donovan LE, Corcoy R, et al. Continuous glucose monitoring in pregnant women with type 1 diabetes (CONCEPTT): A multicentre international randomised controlled trial. *Lancet.* 2017 Nov 25;390(10110): 2347–59.

39. Diabetes in pregnancy (QS109) (accessed 1/3/23). www.nice.org.uk/guid ance/qs109.

40. Difference between a flash glucose monitor and a CGM. [Internet]. [cited 2023 May 25]. www.diabetes.org.uk/guide-to-diabetes/diabetes-technol ogy/flash-glucose-monitors-and-continuous-glucose-monitors#:~: text=Difference%20between%20a%20flash%20glucose,you%20get% 20your%20sugar%20readings.

41. Zhang M, Zhou Y, Zhong J, et al. Current guidelines on the management of gestational diabetes mellitus: A content analysis and appraisal. *BMC Pregnancy Childbirth.* 2019;19(1):200.

42. Recommendations | Diabetes in pregnancy: Management from preconception to the postnatal period | Guidance | NICE [Internet]. [cited 2020 Jan 10]. www.nice.org.uk/guidance/ng3/chapter/1-Recommendations# antenatal-care-for-women-with-diabetes-2.

43. Eyal S, Easterling TR, Carr D, et al. Pharmacokinetics of metformin during pregnancy. *Drug Metab Dispos.* 2010 May;38(5):833–40. https://doi.org/ 10.1124/dmd.109.031245. Epub 2010 Jan 29. PMID: 20118196.

44. Gilbert C, Valois M, Koren G. Pregnancy outcome after first-trimester exposure to metformin: A meta-analysis. *Fertil Steril.* 2006;86(3):658–63.

45. Cassina M, Donà M, Di Gianantonio E, et al. First-trimester exposure to metformin and risk of birth defects: A systematic review and meta-analysis. *Hum Reprod Update.* 2014;20(5):656–69.

46. Elmaraezy A, Abushouk AI, Emara A, et al. Effect of metformin on maternal and neonatal outcomes in pregnant obese non-diabetic women: A meta-analysis. *Int J Reprod Biomed Yazd Iran.* 2017;15(8):461–70.

47. Rowan JA, Hague WM, Gao W, et al.; MiG Trial Investigators. Metformin versus insulin for the treatment of gestational diabetes. *N Engl J Med.* 2008 May 8;358(19):2003–15.

48. SMFM Statement: Pharmacological treatment of gestational diabetes. *Am J Obstet Gynecol.* 2018;218(5):B2–4.

49. Kjos SL, Schaefer-Graf UM. Modified therapy for gestational diabetes using high-risk and low-risk fetal abdominal circumference growth to

select strict versus relaxed maternal glycemic targets. *Diabetes Care.* 2007;30(2):S200–05.

50. Toledano Y, Hadar E, Hod M. Pharmacotherapy for hyperglycemia in pregnancy – The new insulins. *Diabetes Res Clin Pract.* 2018;145:59–66.

51. Pöyhönen-Alho M, Rönnemaa T, Saltevo J, et al. Use of insulin glargine during pregnancy. *Acta Obstet Gynecol Scand.* 2007;86(10):1171–74.

52. Pantalone KM, Faiman C, Olansky L. Insulin glargine use during pregnancy. *Endocr Pract Off J Am Coll Endocrinol Am Assoc Clin Endocrinol.* 2011; 17(3):448–55.

53. Lepercq J, Lin J, Hall GC, et al. Meta-analysis of maternal and neonatal outcomes associated with the use of insulin glargine versus NPH insulin during pregnancy. *Obstet Gynecol Int.* 2012;2012:649070.

54. TOUJEO (insulin glargine injection) U-300 [prescribing information]. Bridgewater, NJ: Sanofi-Aventis, 02/2015.

55. Lee TTM, Collett C, Bergford S, et al. AiDAPT Collaborative Group. Automated insulin delivery in women with pregnancy complicated by type 1 diabetes. *N Engl J Med.* 2023 Oct 26;389(17):1566–78.

56. Bibbins-Domingo K, Grossman DC, et al. Folic acid supplementation for the prevention of neural tube defects: US Preventive Services Task Force Recommendation Statement. *JAMA* 2017;317(2):183.

57. Diabetes Control and Complications Trial Research Group. Effect of pregnancy on microvascular complications in the diabetes control and complications trial. The Diabetes Control and Complications Trial Research Group. *Diabetes Care.* 2000;23(8):1084–91.

58. Vestgaard M, Ringholm L, Laugesen CS, et al. Pregnancy-induced sight-threatening diabetic retinopathy in women with Type 1 diabetes. *Diabet Med J Br Diabet Assoc.* 2010;27(4):431–35.

59. Rasmussen KL, Laugesen CS, Ringholm L, et al. Progression of diabetic retinopathy during pregnancy in women with type 2 diabetes. *Diabetologia.* 2010;53(6):1076–83.

60. Moloney JB, Drury MI. The effect of pregnancy on the natural course of diabetic retinopathy. *Am J Ophthalmol.* 1982;93(6):745–56.

61. Bullo M, Tschumi S, Bucher BS, et al. Pregnancy outcome following exposure to angiotensin-converting enzyme inhibitors or angiotensin receptor antagonists: A systematic review. *Hypertension.* 2012;60(2):444–50.

62. Podymow T, Joseph G. Preconception and pregnancy management of women with diabetic nephropathy on angiotensin converting enzyme inhibitors. *Clin Nephrol.* 2015;83(2):73–79.

63. American Academy of Pediatrics Committee on Drugs. Transfer of drugs and other chemicals into human milk. *Pediatrics.* 2001;108(3):776–89.

64. Elkayam U, Goland S, Pieper PG, et al. High-risk cardiac disease in pregnancy: Part I. *J Am Coll Cardiol.* 2016;68(4):396–410.

65. ACOG Practice Bulletin No. 190: Gestational Diabetes Mellitus. *Obstet Gynecol.* 2018 Feb;131(2):e49.

66. Hypertension in pregnancy: Diagnosis and management [NG133]. www .nice.org.uk/guidance/ng133.

67. Goldberg AS, Hegele RA. Severe hypertriglyceridemia in pregnancy. *J Clin Endocrinol Metab.* 2012;97(8):2589–96.

68. Alvarez-Marfany M, Roman SH, Drexler AJ, et al. Long-term prospective study of postpartum thyroid dysfunction in women with insulin dependent diabetes mellitus. *J Clin Endocrinol Metab.* 1994;79(1):10–16.

69. Corbin KD, Driscoll KA, Pratley RE, et al. Obesity in type 1 diabetes: Pathophysiology, clinical impact, and mechanisms. *Endocr Rev.* 2018; 39(5):629–63.

70. Metzger, BE, Buchanan, TA, Coustan, DR, et al. Summary and recommendations of the Fifth International Workshop-Conference on Gestational Diabetes Mellitus. *Diabetes Care.* 2007;30(Suppl 2):S251–60.

71. Viana, LV, Gross, JL, Azevedo, MJ. Dietary intervention in patients with gestational diabetes mellitus: A systematic review and meta-analysis of randomized clinical trials on maternal and newborn outcomes. *Diabetes Care.* 2014;37:3345–55.

72. Mikines, KJ, Sonne, B, Farrell, PA, Tronier, B, Galbo, H. Effect of physical exercise on sensitivity and responsiveness to insulin in humans. *Am J Physiol.*1988;254:E248–59.

73. Lee R, Thain S, Tan LK et al. IPRAMHO Exercise in Pregnancy Committee. Asia-Pacific consensus on physical activity and exercise in pregnancy and the postpartum period. *BMJ Open Sport Exerc Med.* 2021;7: e000967. https://doi.org/10.1136/bmjsem-2020-000967.

74. World Health Organization. *Diagnostic Criteria and Classification of Hyperglycaemia First Detected in Pregnancy.* 2013. http://apps.who.int/ iris/bitstream/10665/85975/1/WHO_NMH_MND_13.2_eng.pdf.

75. International Association of Diabetes and Pregnancy Study Groups Consensus Panel; Metzger BE, Gabbe SG, Persson B, et al. International Association of Diabetes and Pregnancy Study Groups recommendations on the diagnosis and classification of hyperglycemia in pregnancy. *Diabetes Care.* 2010 Mar;33(3): 676–82.

76. Diabetes Canada Clinical Practice Guidelines Expert Committee. Diabetes Canada 2018 Clinical Practice Guidelines for the prevention and management of diabetes in Canada. *Can J Diabetes.* 2018;42(Suppl 1):S1–325.

77. ElSayed NA, Aleppo G, Aroda VR, et al. 2. Classification and Diagnosis of Diabetes: Standards of Care in Diabetes – 2023. *Diabetes Care*. 2023 Jan 1;46(Suppl 1):S19–40.

78. Chong YS, Cai S, Lin H, et al. Ethnic differences translate to inadequacy of high-risk screening for gestational diabetes mellitus in an Asian population: A cohort study. *BMC Pregnancy Childbirth*. 2014 Oct 2;14:345.

79. HAPO Study Cooperative Research Group. Hyperglycemia and Adverse Pregnancy Outcome (HAPO) Study: Associations with neonatal anthropometrics. *Diabetes*. 2009 Feb;58(2):453–59.

80. 2014 ADIPSGDM Guidelines V18.11.2014_000 [Internet]. [cited 2023 1 March]. www.adips.org/downloads/2014ADIPSGDMGuidelines V18.11.2014_000.pdf.

81. Hod M, Kapur A, Sacks DA, et al. The International Federation of Gynecology and Obstetrics (FIGO) initiative on gestational diabetes mellitus: A pragmatic guide for diagnosis, management, and care. *Int J Gynaecol Obstet*. 2015 Oct;131(Suppl 3):S173–211.

82. Goldberg A, Ursing C, Ekéus C, Wiberg-Itzel E. Swedish guidelines for type 1 diabetes and pregnancy outcomes: A nationwide descriptive study of consensus and adherence. *Primary Care Diabetes*. 2021 Dec;15(6):1040–51.

83. Pregnancy and Insulin Resistance | Metabolic Syndrome and Related Disorders [Internet]. [cited 2020 Jan 10]. www.liebertpub.com/doi/ 10.1089/met.2006.4.149.

84. Hernandez TL, Friedman JE, Van Pelt RE, et al. Patterns of glycemia in normal pregnancy. *Diabetes Care*. 2011;34(7):1660–68.

85. Willman SP, Leveno KJ, Guzick DS, et al. Glucose threshold for macrosomia in pregnancy complicated by diabetes. *Am J Obstet Gynecol*. 1986;154(2):470–75.

86. Veciana MD, Toohey JS. Postprandial versus preprandial blood glucose monitoring in women with gestational diabetes mellitus requiring insulin therapy. *N Engl J Med*. 1995;333(19):5.

87. Crowther CA, Samuel D, Hughes R, et al. Tighter or less tight glycaemic targets for women with gestational diabetes mellitus for reducing maternal and perinatal morbidity: A stepped-wedge, cluster-randomised trial. *PLoS Med*. 2022 Sep;19(9):e1004087.

88. Landon MB, Carpenter MW, Wapner RJ, et al. A multicenter, randomized trial of treatment for mild gestational diabetes. *N Engl J Med*. 2009;361-(14):1339–48.

89. Martis R, Crowther CA, Shepherd E, et al. Treatments for women with gestational diabetes mellitus: An overview of Cochrane systematic reviews. *Cochrane Database Syst Rev*. 2018 Aug 14;8(8):CD012327.

90. Abell SK, Boyle JA, Earnest A, et al. Impact of different glycaemic treatment targets on pregnancy outcomes in gestational diabetes. *Diabet Med.* 2019 Feb;36(2):177–83.

91. Diabetes Canada Clinical Practice Guidelines Expert Committee, Feig DS, Berger H, et al. Diabetes and pregnancy. *Can J Diabetes.* 2018 Apr;42(Suppl 1):S255–82.

92. Gabbe SG, Mestman JH, Hibbard LT. Maternal mortality in diabetes mellitus: An 18-year survey. *Obstet Gynecol.* 1976;(48):549–51.

93. American College of Obstetricians and Gynecologists' Committee on Practice Bulletins – Obstetrics. ACOG Practice Bulletin No. 201: Pregestational Diabetes Mellitus. *Obstet Gynecol.* 2018 Dec;132(6): e228–48.

94. Raman P, Shepherd E, Dowswell T, Middleton P, Crowther CA. Different methods and settings for glucose monitoring for gestational diabetes during pregnancy. *Cochrane Database Syst Rev.* 2017 Oct 29;10(10): CD011069.

95. Jovanovic-Peterson L, Peterson CM, Reed GF, et al. Maternal postprandial glucose levels and infant birth weight: The Diabetes in Early Pregnancy Study. The National Institute of Child Health and Human Development – Diabetes in Early Pregnancy Study. *Am J Obstet Gynecol.* 1991;164(1 Pt 1):103–11.

96. Manderson JG, Patterson CC, Hadden DR, et al. Preprandial versus postprandial blood glucose monitoring in type 1 diabetic pregnancy: A randomized controlled clinical trial. *Am J Obstet Gynecol.* 2003;189(2):507–12.

97. Ben-Haroush A, Yogev Y, Chen R, et al. The postprandial glucose profile in the diabetic pregnancy. *Am J Obstet Gynecol.* 2004;191(2):576–81.

98. Kerssen A, de Valk HW, Visser GHA. Day-to-day glucose variability during pregnancy in women with Type 1 diabetes mellitus: Glucose profiles measured with the Continuous Glucose Monitoring System. *Br J Obstet Gynaecol.* 2004;111(9):919–24.

99. Sivan E, Weisz B, Homko CJ, et al. One or two hours postprandial glucose measurements: Are they the same? *Am J Obstet Gynecol.* 2001;185 (3):604–07.

100. Stanley K, Magides A, Arnot M, et al. Delayed gastric emptying as a factor in delayed postprandial glycaemic response in pregnancy. *Br J Obstet Gynaecol.* 1995;102(4):288–91.

101. Hewapathirana NM, O'Sullivan E, Murphy HR. Role of continuous glucose monitoring in the management of diabetic pregnancy. *Curr Diab Rep.* 2013;13(1):34–42.

102. Yogev Y, Ben-Haroush A, Chen R, et al. Continuous glucose monitoring for treatment adjustment in diabetic pregnancies – A pilot study. *Diabet Med J Br Diabet Assoc.* 2003;20(7):558–62.

103. Bidonde J, Fagerlund BC, Frønsdal KB, et al. FreeStyle Libre Flash Glucose Self-Monitoring System: A Single-Technology Assessment [Internet]. Oslo, Norway: Knowledge Centre for the Health Services at The Norwegian Institute of Public Health (NIPH); 2017 Aug 21. Report from the Norwegian Institute of Public Health No. 2017–07.

104. Leelarathna L, Wilmot EG. Flash forward: A review of flash glucose monitoring. *Diabet Med J Br Diabet Assoc.* 2018;35(4):472–82.

105. Snapshot [Internet]. [cited 2023 Feb 13]. www.freestylelibre.co.uk/libre/discover/diabetes-management-pregnancy.html.

106. Blum A. Freestyle Libre Glucose Monitoring System. *Clin Diabetes.* 2018 Apr;36(2):203–04. https://doi.org/10.2337/cd17-0130.

107. Gatti M, Amato AML, Bruttomesso D. FreeStyle Libre flash glucose monitoring system in pregnant woman with type 1 diabetes: a focus on accuracy. *Acta Diabetol.* 2019;56(8):969–70.

108. Gallagher EJ, Le Roith D, Bloomgarden Z. Review of hemoglobin A(1c) in the management of diabetes. *J Diabetes.* 2009;1(1):9–17.

109. Nielsen LR, Ekbom P, Damm P, et al. HbA1c Levels Are Significantly Lower in Early and Late Pregnancy. *Diabetes Care.* 2004;27(5):1200–01.

110. Jovanovic L, Savas H, Mehta M, et al. Frequent monitoring of A1C during pregnancy as a treatment tool to guide therapy. *Diabetes Care.* 2011;34(1):53–54.

111. Combs CA, Gunderson E, Kitzmiller JL, Gavin LA, Main EK. Relationship of fetal macrosomia to maternal postprandial glucose control during pregnancy. *Diabetes Care.* 1992 Oct;15(10):1251–57.

112. Suhonen L, Hiilesmaa V, Teramo K. Glycaemic control during early pregnancy and fetal malformations in women with type I diabetes mellitus. *Diabetologia.* 2000;43(1):79–82.

113. Guerin A, Nisenbaum R, Ray JG. Use of maternal GHb concentration to estimate the risk of congenital anomalies in the offspring of women with prepregnancy diabetes. *Diabetes Care.* 2007;30(7):1920–25.

114. Murphy HR, Howgate C, O'Keefe J, et al. Characteristics and outcomes of pregnant women with type 1 or type 2 diabetes: A 5-year national population-based cohort study. *Lancet Diabetes Endocrinol.* 2021 Mar; 9(3):153–64.

115. Poo ZX, Wright A, Ruochen D, Singh R. Optimal first trimester HbA1c threshold to identify Singaporean women at risk of gestational diabetes mellitus and adverse pregnancy outcomes: A pilot study. *Obstet Med.* 2019

Jun;12(2):79–84. https://doi.org/10.1177/1753495X18795984. Epub 2018 Nov 15. PMID: 31217812; PMCID: PMC6560840.

116. Combs CA, Gunderson E, Kitzmiller JL, et al. Relationship of fetal macrosomia to maternal postprandial glucose control during pregnancy. *Diabetes Care*. 1992;15(10):1251–57.

117. Bennett SN, Tita A, Owen J, Biggio JR, Harper LM. Assessing White's classification of pregestational diabetes in a contemporary diabetic population. *Obstet Gynecol*. 2015 May;125(5):1217–23.

118. Sibai BM, Caritis S, Hauth J, et al. Risks of preeclampsia and adverse neonatal outcomes among women with pregestational diabetes mellitus. National Institute of Child Health and Human Development Network of Maternal–Fetal Medicine Units. *Am J Obstet Gynecol*. 2000 Feb;182 (2):364–69.

119. Roberge S, Bujold E, Nicolaides KH. Aspirin for the prevention of preterm and term preeclampsia: Systematic review and metaanalysis. *Am J Obstet Gynecol*. 2018;218(3):287–293.e1.

120. Dietary Reference Intakes Tables and Application: Health and Medicine Division [Internet]. [cited 2020 Jan 14]. http://nationalacademies.org/ hmd/Activities/Nutrition/SummaryDRIs/DRI-Tables.aspx.

121. Louie JCY, Brand-Miller JC, Moses RG. Carbohydrates, glycemic index, and pregnancy outcomes in gestational diabetes. *Curr Diab Rep*. 2013 Feb 1;13(1):6–11.

122. Yee LM, Cheng YW, Inturrisi M, Caughey AB. Effect of gestational weight gain on perinatal outcomes in women with type 2 diabetes mellitus using the 2009 Institute of Medicine guidelines. *Am J Obstet Gynecol*. 2011 Sep;205(3):257.e1–6.

123. Harper LM, Shanks AL, Odibo AO, et al. Gestational weight gain in insulin-resistant pregnancies. *J Perinatol*. 2013 Dec;33(12):929–33.

124. Institute of Medicine (US) and National Research Council (US) Committee to Reexamine IOM Pregnancy Weight Guidelines. Weight Gain During Pregnancy: Reexamining the Guidelines [Internet]. Rasmussen KM, Yaktine AL. (eds.). Washington (DC): National Academies Press (US), 2009 [cited 2023 Mar 2]. (The National Academies Collection: Reports funded by National Institutes of Health). www.ncbi.nlm.nih.gov/books/ NBK32813/.

125. Peters TM, Brazeau AS. Exercise in pregnant women with diabetes. *Curr Diab Rep*. 2019 Aug 6;19(9):80.

126. Morrison JL, Hodgson LA, Lim LL, et al. Diabetic retinopathy in pregnancy: A review. *Clin Experiment Ophthalmol*. 2016;44(4):321–34.

127. Polizzi S, Mahajan VB. Intravitreal anti-VEGF injections in pregnancy: Case series and review of literature. *J Ocul Pharmacol Ther.* 2015;31 (10):605–10.

128. Bramham K. Diabetic nephropathy and pregnancy. *Semin Nephrol.* 2017;37(4):362–69.

129. Cundy T, Slee F, Gamble G, et al. Hypertensive disorders of pregnancy in women with Type 1 and Type 2 diabetes. *Diabet Med J Br Diabet Assoc.* 2002;19(6):482–89.

130. Yogev Y, Xenakis EMJ, Langer O. The association between preeclampsia and the severity of gestational diabetes: the impact of glycemic control. *Am J Obstet Gynecol.* 2004 Nov;191(5):1655–60.

131. Ostlund, I, Hanson, U, Bjorklund, A, et al. Maternal and fetal outcomes if gestational impaired glucose tolerance is not treated. *Diabetes Care.* 2003; 26: 2107–11.

132. Weissgerber TL, Mudd LM. Preeclampsia and diabetes. *Curr Diab Rep.* 2015;15(3):9.

133. Persson M, Norman M, Hanson U. Obstetric and perinatal outcomes in type 1 diabetic pregnancies: A large, population-based study. *Diabetes Care.* 2009;32(11):2005–09.

134. Knight KM, Thornburg LL, Pressman EK. Pregnancy outcomes in type 2 diabetic patients as compared with type 1 diabetic patients and nondiabetic controls. J Reprod Med. 2012;57(9–10):397–404.

135. Montoro MN, Myers VP, Mestman JH, et al. Outcome of pregnancy in diabetic ketoacidosis. *Am J Perinatol.* 1993;10(1):17–20.

136. Rougerie M, Czuzoj-Shulman N, Abenhaim HA. Diabetic ketoacidosis among pregnant and non-pregnant women: A comparison of morbidity and mortality. *J Matern Fetal Neonatal Med.* 2019;32(16):2649–52.

137. Jaber JF, Standley M, Reddy R. Euglycemic diabetic ketoacidosis in pregnancy: A case report and review of current literature. *Case Rep Crit Care.* 2019;2019:8769714.

138. Kamalakannan D, Baskar V, Barton DM, et al. Diabetic ketoacidosis in pregnancy. *Postgrad Med J.* 2003;79(934):454–57.

139. Diguisto C, Strachan MWJ, Churchill D, Ayman G, Knight M. A study of diabetic ketoacidosis in the pregnant population in the United Kingdom: Investigating the incidence, aetiology, management and outcomes. *Diabet Med.* 2022 Apr;39(4):e14743.

140. Ng YHG, Ee TX, Kanagalingam D, et al. Resolution of severe fetal distress following treatment of maternal diabetic ketoacidosis. *BMJ Case Rep.* 2018;2018:bcr2017221325.

141. Coetzee EJ, Jackson WP, Berman PA. Ketonuria in pregnancy – with special reference to calorie-restricted food intake in obese diabetics. *Diabetes.* 1980 Mar;29(3):177–81.

142. Evers IM, ter Braak EWMT, de Valk HW, et al. Risk indicators predictive for severe hypoglycemia during the first trimester of type 1 diabetic pregnancy. *Diabetes Care.* 2002 Mar;25(3):554–59.

143. Kimmerle R, Heinemann L, Delecki A, Berger M. Severe hypoglycemia incidence and predisposing factors in 85 pregnancies of type I diabetic women. *Diabetes Care.* 1992 Aug;15(8):1034–37.

144. Ringholm L, Pedersen-Bjergaard U, Thorsteinsson B, Damm P, Mathiesen ER. Hypoglycaemia during pregnancy in women with type 1 diabetes. *Diabet Med.* 2012;29:558–66.

145. Leinonen PJ, Hiilesmaa VK, Kaaja RJ, Teramo KA. Maternal mortality in type 1 diabetes. *Diabetes Care.* 2001 Aug;24(8):1501–02.

146. Kitzmiller JL, Block JM, Brown FM, et al. Managing preexisting diabetes for pregnancy: Summary of evidence and consensus recommendations for care. *Diabetes Care.* 2008;31:1060–79.

147. Sharpe PB, Chan A, Haan EA, Hiller JE. Maternal diabetes and congenital anomalies in South Australia 1986–2000: A population-based cohort study. *Birth Defects Res A Clin Mol Teratol.* 2005;73:605–11.

148. Garner P. Type I diabetes mellitus and pregnancy. *Lancet.* 1995;346:157–61.

149. Berk MA, Mimouni F, Miodovnik M, Hertzberg V, Valuck J. Macrosomia in infants of insulin-dependent diabetic mothers. *Pediatrics.* 1989;83:1029–34.

150. Farrell T, Neale L, Cundy T. Congenital anomalies in the offspring of women with type 1, type 2 and gestational diabetes. *Diabet Med.* 2002;19:322–26.

151. Reece EA, Homko CJ. Why do diabetic women deliver malformed infants? *Clin Obstet Gynecol.* 2000;43:32–45.

152. Towner D, Kjos SL, Leung B, et al. Congenital malformations in pregnancies complicated by NIDDM. *Diabetes Care.* 1995;18:1446–51.

153. Macfarlane CM, Tsakalakos, N. The extended Pedersen hypothesis. *Clin Physiol Biochem.* 1988;6:68–73.

154. Nesbitt TS, Gilbert WM, Herrchen B. Shoulder dystocia and associated risk factors with macrosomic infants born in California. *Am J Obstet Gynecol.* 1998;179:476–80.

155. Mollberg M, Hagberg H, Bager B, Lilja H, Ladfors L. High birthweight and shoulder dystocia: The strongest risk factors for obstetrical brachial plexus palsy in a Swedish population-based study. *Acta Obstet Gynecol Scand.* 2005;84:654–59.

156. Peck RW, Price DE, Lang GD, MacVicar J, Hearnshaw JR. Birthweight of babies born to mothers with type 1 diabetes: Is it related to blood glucose control in the first trimester? *Diabet Med.* 1991;8:258–62.

157. Bochner CJ, Medearis AL, Williams J, et al. Early third-trimester ultrasound screening in gestational diabetes to determine the risk of macrosomia and labor dystocia at term. *Am J Obstet Gynecol.* 1987;157:703–08.

158. Hawthorne G, Robson S, Ryall EA, et al. Prospective population based survey of outcome of pregnancy in diabetic women: Results of the Northern Diabetic Pregnancy Audit, 1994. *BMJ.* 1997 Aug 2;315(7103):279–81. https://doi.org/10.1136/bmj.315.7103.279.

159. Jabak S, Hameed A. Continuous intrapartum fetal monitoring in gestational diabetes, where is the evidence? *J Matern Fetal Neonatal Med.* 2022 Nov;35(22):4354–57. https://doi.org/10.1080/14767058.2020.1849117.

160. Pietryga M, Brazert J, Wender-Ozegowska E, et al. Abnormal uterine Doppler is related to vasculopathy in pregestational diabetes mellitus. *Circulation.* 2005 Oct 18;112(16):2496–500.

161. Wager J, Fredholm B, Lunell NO, Persson B. Metabolic and circulatory effects of intravenous and oral salbutamol in late pregnancy in diabetic and non-diabetic women. *Acta Obstet Gynecol Scand Suppl.* 1982;108:41–46.

162. Mathiesen ER, Christensen AB, Hellmuth E, et al. Insulin dose during glucocorticoid treatment for fetal lung maturation in diabetic pregnancy: Test of an algorithm. *Acta Obstet Gynecol Scand.* 2002;81:835–39.

163. Thiebaugeorges O, Guyard-Boileau B. Obstetrical care in gestational diabetes and management of preterm labour. *Diabetes Metab.* 2010;36(6 Pt 2):672–81.

164. Liggins Institute. [Internet]. [cited 2023 May 2023]. www.ligginstrials .org/Precede_Test/.

165. Garabedian, C, Deruelle, P. Delivery (timing, route, peripartum glycemic control) in women with gestational diabetes mellitus. *Diabetes Metab.* 2010; 36: 515–21.

166. Boulvain M, Senat M-V, Perrotin F, et al. Induction of labour versus expectant management for large-for-date fetuses: A randomised controlled trial. *Lancet Lond Engl.* 2015;385(9987):2600–05.

167. Donnelly V, Foran A, Murphy J, et al. Neonatal brachial plexus palsy: An unpredictable injury. *Am J Obstet Gynecol.* 2002;187:1209–12.

168. Montgomery (Appellant) v Lanarkshire Health Board (Respondent) (Scotland) [2015] UKSC 11. 2015.

169. Cundy T, Gamble G, Townend K, et al. Perinatal mortality in type 2 diabetes mellitus. *Diabet Med.* 2000;17:33–39.

170. Mitanchez D. Fetal and neonatal complications in gestational diabetes: Perinatal mortality, congenital malformations, macrosomia, shoulder dystocia, birth injuries, neonatal complications. *Diabetes Metab.* 2010;36: 617–27.

171. Golde SH, Good-Anderson B, Montoro M, et al. Insulin requirements during labor: A reappraisal. *Am J Obstet Gynecol.* 1982;144(5):556–59.

172. Kenepp, NB, Kumar, S, Shelley, WC, et al. Fetal and neonatal hazards of maternal hydration with 5% dextrose before caesarean section. *Lancet.* 1982;1:1150–52.

173. Anderson PO. Treating diabetes during breastfeeding. *Breastfeed Med.* 2018;13(4):237–39.

174. Kim C, Newton KM, Knopp RH. Gestational diabetes and the incidence of type 2 diabetes: A systematic review. *Diabetes Care.* 2002;25:1862–68.

175. WHO, Department of Reproductive Health and Research. Medical Eligibility Criteria for Contraceptive Use, 5th edn. (2015). www.who .int/publications/i/item/9789241549158

176. WHO Medical Eligibility Criteria for Contraceptive Use; Geneva: 2015. www.ncbi.nlm.nih.gov/pmc/articles/PMC5683149/table/t3-oajc-7-011/ ?report=objectonly.

177. Cordero, L, Treuer, SH, Landon, MB, Gabbe, SG. Management of infants of diabetic mothers. *Arch Pediatr Adolesc Med.* 1998;152:249–54.

178. Sobngwi E, Boudou P, Mauvais-Jarvis F, et al. Effect of a diabetic environment in utero on predisposition to type 2 diabetes. *Lancet.* 2003;361: 1861–65.

179. Clausen TD, Mathiesen ER, Hansen T, et al. Overweight and the metabolic syndrome in adult offspring of women with diet-treated gestational diabetes mellitus or type 1 diabetes. *J Clin Endocrinol Metab.* 2009;94:2464–70.

180. Tsang RC, Ballard J, Braun C. The infant of the diabetic mother: Today and tomorrow. *Clin Obstet Gynecol.* 1981;24:125–47.

181. Katz L, Tsang RC. Hypocalcemia in infants of diabetic mothers. *J Pediatr.* 1972;81:633–34.

182. Mimouni F, Tsang RC, Hertzberg VS, Miodovnik M. Polycythemia, hypomagnesemia, and hypocalcemia in infants of diabetic mothers. *Am J Dis Child.* 1986;140(8):798–800. https://doi.org/10.1001/archpedi.1986.021402 20080037.

183. Landon MB. Is there a benefit to the treatment of mild gestational diabetes mellitus? *Am J Obstet Gynecol.* 2010;202:649–53.

184. Damm P. Future risk of diabetes in mother and child after gestational diabetes mellitus. *Int J Gynaecol Obstet.* 2009 Mar;104(Suppl 1):S25–26.

185. Sheiner E. Gestational diabetes mellitus: Long-term consequences for the mother and child grand challenge: How to move on towards secondary prevention? *Front Clin Diabetes Healthc.* 2020 Nov 4;1:546256.

186. Metzger BE. Long-term outcomes in mothers diagnosed with gestational diabetes mellitus and their offspring. *Clin Obstet Gynecol.* 2007 Dec;50(4): 972–79.

187. O'Reilly SL. Prevention of diabetes after gestational diabetes: better translation of nutrition and lifestyle messages needed. *Healthcare (Basel).* 2014 Nov 21;2(4):468–91. https://doi.org/10.3390/healthcare2040468.

188. Barker DJ. The fetal and infant origins of adult disease. *BMJ.* 1990 Nov 17;301(6761):1111.

189. Gluckman PD, Hanson MA. Living with the past: Evolution, development, and patterns of disease. *Science.* 2004 Sep 17;305(5691):1733–36.

Cambridge Elements ☰

High-Risk Pregnancy: Management Options

Professor David James
Emeritus Professor, University of Nottingham, UK

David James was Professor of Fetomaternal Medicine at the University of Nottingham from 1992–2009. The post involved clinical service, especially the management of high-risk pregnancies, guideline development, research and teaching and NHS management. From 2009–14 he was Clinical Director of Women's Health at the National Centre for Clinical Excellence for Women's and Children's Health. He was also Clinical Lead for the RCOG/RCM/eLfH eFM E-Learning Project. He is a recognised authority on the management of problem/complicated pregnancies with over 200 peer-reviewed publications. He has published 16 books, the best-known being *High-Risk Pregnancy: Management Options*.

Professor Philip Steer
Emeritus Professor, Imperial College, London, UK

Philip Steer is Emeritus Professor of Obstetrics at Imperial College London, having been appointed Professor in 1989. He was a consultant obstetrician for 35 years. He was Editor-in-Chief of *BJOG – An International Journal of Obstetrics and Gynaecology* – from 2005–2012, and is now Editor Emeritus. He has published more than 150 peer-reviewed research papers, 109 reviews and editorials and 66 book chapters/books, the best known and most successful being *High-Risk Pregnancy: Management Options*. The fifth edition was published in 2018. He has been President of the British Association of Perinatal Medicine and President of the Section of Obstetrics and Gynaecology of the Royal Society of Medicine. He is an honorary fellow of the College of Obstetricians and Gynaecologists of South Africa, and of the American Gynecological & Obstetrical Society.

Professor Carl Weiner
Creighton University School of Medicine, Phoenix, AZ, USA

Carl Weiner is presently Head of Maternal Fetal Medicine for the CommonSpirit Health System, Arizona, Director of Maternal Fetal Medicine, Dignity St Joseph's Hospital, Professor, Obstetrics and Gynecology, Creighton School of Medicine, Phoenix, and Professor, College of Health Solutions, Arizona State University. He is the former Krantz Professor and Chair of Obstetrics and Gynecology, Division Head Maternal Fetal Medicine and Professor Molecular and Integrative Physiology at the University of Kansas School of Medicine, Kansas City, KS and the Crenshaw Professor and Chair of Obstetrics, Gynecology and Reproductive Biology, Division Head Maternal Fetal Medicine, and Professor of Physiology at the University of Maryland School of Medicine, Baltimore. Dr Weiner has published more than 265 peer-reviewed research articles and authored/edited 18 textbooks including *High-Risk Pregnancy: Management Options*. His research was extramurally funded for more than 30 years without interruption.

Professor Stephen Robson
Newcastle University, UK

Stephen C. Robson is Emeritus Professor of Fetal Medicine for the Population and Health Sciences Institute at The Medical School, Newcastle University. He is also a Consultant in Fetal Medicine for Newcastle upon Tyne Hospitals NHS Foundation Trust. He has published over 400 peer-reviewed articles and edited several; books, the highly successful being *High Risk Pregnancy: Management Options*. The fifth edition was published in 2018. He has been President of the British Maternal and Fetal Medicine.

About the Series

Most pregnancies are uncomplicated. However, for some ('high-risk' pregnancies) an adverse outcome for the mother and/or the baby is more likely. Each Element in the series covers a specific high-risk problem/condition in pregnancy. The risks of the condition will be listed followed by an evidence-based review of the management options. Once the series is complete, the Elements will be collated and printed in a sixth edition of *High-Risk Pregnancy: Management Options*.

Cambridge Elements ≡

High-Risk Pregnancy: Management Options

Elements in the Series

A full series listing is available at: www.cambridge.org/EHRP

Printed in the United States
by Baker & Taylor Publisher Services